WHAT YOU MUST KNOW ABOUT
EYESTRAIN

Other Works by Dr. Jeff Anshel

Smart Medicine for Your Eyes

*What You Must Know About
Age-Related Macular Degeneration*

What You Must Know About Dry Eye

*What You Must Know About
Food and Supplements for Optimal Vision Care*

WHAT YOU MUST KNOW ABOUT
EYESTRAIN

JEFFREY ANSHEL, OD

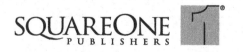

SQUAREONE
PUBLISHERS

The information and advice contained in this book are based upon the research and the personal and professional experiences of the author. They are not intended as a substitute for consulting with a healthcare professional. The publisher and author are not responsible for any adverse effects or consequences resulting from the use of any of the suggestions, preparations, or procedures discussed in this book. All matters pertaining to your physical health should be supervised by a healthcare professional. It is a sign of wisdom, not cowardice, to seek a second or third opinion.

Cover Designer: Jeannie Rosado
Typesetter: Gary A. Rosenberg

Square One Publishers
115 Herricks Road
Garden City Park, NY 11040
(516) 535-2010 • (877) 900-BOOK
www.squareonepublishers.com

Library of Congress Cataloging-in-Publication Data
Names: Anshel, Jeffrey, author.
Title: What you must know about eyestrain / Jeffrey Anshel, OD.
Description: Garden City Park, NY : Square One Publishers, [2022] |
    Includes bibliographical references and index.
Identifiers: LCCN 2021041081 (print) | LCCN 2021041082 (ebook) | ISBN
    9780757005015 (paperback) | ISBN 9780757055010 (ebook)
Subjects: LCSH: Eyestrain.
Classification: LCC RE48 .A57 2022 (print) | LCC RE48 (ebook) | DDC
    617.7—dc23
LC record available at https://lccn.loc.gov/2021041081
LC ebook record available at https://lccn.loc.gov/2021041082

Printed in the United States of America

10   9   8   7   6   5   4   3   2

Contents

This book is dedicated to my son, Casey,
who continues to inspire me to be
the best person I can be.

This book has been printed on cream-colored paper
to reduce eyestrain as you read.

Introduction

Do your eyes feel tired at the end of the day? Do they feel dry after you've spent a few hours on the computer? Are they red and irritated? Is your vision fluctuating? Do you get a headache after watching a movie or reading a book? If you answered yes to any of the previous questions, you are likely experiencing what millions of people here and around the world experience every day: eyestrain. Eyestrain is one of the most common problems associated with our changing visual demands as well as our modern lifestyles.

Eyestrain is not necessarily a vision-threatening disease, but it can sure make your life miserable. Whether you are trying to get your work done on a deadline or just texting your friends in the evenings, eyestrain can create havoc in your life. It's simply no fun. Our eyes are our main way to interact with the world, and not only must they see clearly but also function smoothly to allow crisp and comfortable vision. This book is designed to help you to correct or avoid eyestrain so you can maintain proper vision. It will guide you along a path of discovery to determine the sources of eyestrain in your life and how to address them successfully. Some of the solutions to eyestrain might be to correct your eyeglass prescription, change your contact lenses, use a computer the correct way, or eat the right diet to support healthy eyes.

This book is divided into eleven chapters. Chapter 1 covers the anatomy of the eye and the visual system, so you can get a sense of how things need to work to allow you to see clearly. Chapter 2 looks at the definition of eyestrain and what the symptoms of this condition might be, as well as how this problem might be alleviated. Chapter 3 explains how our eyes work when they look at digital images, which include images on monitors, laptops, cell phones, smart watches, and any other device that displays images as a combination of pixels. Given the enormous amount of time we spend viewing digital images, this chapter goes in depth to cover many aspects of this issue at work and in social activities. Chapter 4 describes how our eyes work when they read text on paper, which can still lead to symptoms of eyestrain. In Chapter 5, we discuss eyeglass lenses, how they may be inappropriate for different types of viewing, and how this mismatch can lead to significant eyestrain.

Lighting is a critical part of how we see in various situations, and it differs when we view digital images as opposed to printed text. There are a myriad of different lighting sources, so in Chapter 6 we cover several common lighting conditions and show how to relieve eyestrain with proper lighting. Stress is a significant part of eyestrain, so Chapter 7 lists a number of different stressful situations in which we often use our eyes. As we age, the functioning of our eyes changes, so simply getting older can cause various eyestrain conditions. In Chapter 8, we cover the various changes that occur with age in the visual system, and how they can potentially lead to eyestrain.

Since the eyes are part of the body, we must consider the choices we make that affect our bodies. If our diet or lifestyle interferes with proper bodily function, then our eyes may also be affected. Chapter 9 reviews the different nutrients that support eye health and can help to relieve eyestrain as well. In addition, many of us take medications for various medical conditions. These medications can have significant side effects, many of which can affect the function of the eyes and visual system. In Chapter 10, we look at how these side effects can affect vision.

In Chapter 11, we offer some general eye "exercises" designed to help maintain or improve the functioning of our eyes. (I hesitate to use the term "exercise" without qualification in connection with these techniques, however, as they do not improve muscle strength but rather improve the focusing and coordination of the visual system.)

The book ends with a list of resources that can help you to find the materials and nutritional support sometimes necessary to reduce eyestrain.

If you are one of the millions of people who suffer from eyestrain on a daily—with or without glasses—and think you could never alleviate it, think again. Once you understand the cause of eyestrain and the steps you can take to overcome it, you will have the power to make eyestrain a thing of the past. As you will learn from the chapters that follow, with just a few simple changes, you can make those sore eye pains go away forever.

1

Your Eyes and the Visual System

This book is not designed to be a technical medical synopsis of the anatomy and physiology of the human visual system. To grasp how eyestrain develops, however, you should have some general information of how the eye works in order to have some background with which to make intelligent decisions regarding eyestrain. We will start with some basic eye anatomy, just so you know what's what regarding the parts of the eye. Then you may understand how these parts work together to create this fascinating sense of vision.

LOOK AT YOUR EYES

The eyeball is essentially that—a ball. Its diameter is roughly an inch, and it is about three inches in circumference. The part of the eye that is visible to the world—between the eyelids—is actually only one-sixth of the eye's total surface area. The remaining surface area of the eyeball is hidden behind the eyelids. The outer surface of the eye is divided into two parts: the *sclera* (SKLER-ah), the white part that is the outer covering of the eye, and the *cornea* (KOR-nee-ah), the transparent membrane in front of the eye. (See Figure 1.1 on page 4.)

The cornea, which is steeper in curvature than the sclera, may be difficult to see because it is transparent and backed by the colored *iris* (EYE-ris). You can see the cornea easier if you look at a friend's eye from the side. The cornea serves to protect the eye (it is a very sensitive membrane) and to act as a lens to begin the focusing of light.

3

We traditionally think of the cornea as the first surface that light strikes when entering the eye, however, the light also has to go through the tear layer that covers the front of the eye. Being very thin (much thinner than a human hair), you might not think that it could affect the focusing of the light, but if you have dry (or excessively wet) eyes, you have realized how important an even and uniform tear layer is in the visual process. If the tear film is uneven—too thin or too thick—it will distort the vision and possibly create eyestrain. This fact becomes obvious when you find yourself blinking several times in order to see something clearly, or when you sometimes have to widen your eyelids and hold them open for a few seconds before an image becomes clear. Either situation can lead to eyestrain due to an inadequate tear film.

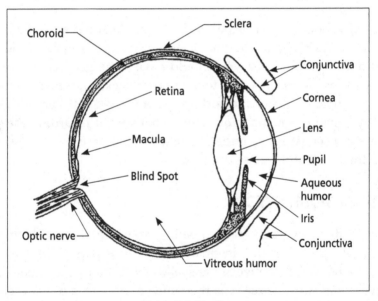

Figure 1.1. The Eye

The sclera is made of tough fibers, which allow it to perform its function of supporting the contents of the eyeball. It has a white appearance because the fibers are light in color, and because it contains very few blood vessels. Just inside the sclera and covering the same area is the *choroid* (KOH-royd), which is the main blood supply to the inner eyeball. Just inside the choroid is the *retina* (RET-in-ah), the nerve membrane that receives the light.

The small but important central area of the retina is called the *macula* (MAC-you-lah). The macula is the area of the retina used for sharp, detailed vision, such as threading a needle or spotting a distant object. The central part of the macula is called the *fovea* (FOE-vee-ah), a small depression in the retina of the eye where visual acuity is highest.

In addition to the blood vessels of the choroid, there are also blood vessels that enter the eye through the optic nerve and lie on the front surface of the retina. They supply nutrition to the retina and other structures inside the eye. These parts all seem to be very basic when you think of what an eye must do. The eye needs protection and support (provided by the sclera), a blood supply (provided by the choroid and through the optic nerve), and a mechanism for seeing (provided by the retina).

When you look at an eye, the first thing you will notice is the iris. If you look closely at an eye, you will see that the iris is enclosed in what is known as a chamber, which is a medical term for a closed space. The iris is surrounded by a watery fluid called the *aqueous* (AY-kwee-us) *humor,* or aqueous fluid. (The term "humor," in this case, does not have anything to do with being funny; it is just the Latin word for fluid.) Just behind the iris is the lens, which facilitates focusing. The lens, also known as the crystalline lens, is transparent and cannot be seen from the outside unless special equipment is used. Behind the lens, and filling the main chamber within the eye, is the *vitreous* (VIT-ree-us) *humor.* The vitreous humor is more gel-like and less watery than the aqueous humor and helps in the support of the retina and other structures.

How the Eye Works

Let's look at the visual process by starting at the beginning. Light enters the eye by passing through the tear layer, the cornea, the aqueous humor, and the pupil. It is focused by the lens and then goes through the vitreous humor and onto the retina. (The retina is actually an extension of the brain, since the nerve fibers from the retina go directly into the brain.)

The light that strikes the retina first stimulates chemical changes in the light-sensitive cells of the retina, known as the *photoreceptors.* There are actually two kinds of photoreceptors: *rods* and *cones.* Rods are long, slender cells that respond to light or dark stimuli and are important to night vision. Cones are cone-shaped cells that respond to color stimuli and therefore are also known as *color receptors.* There are about seventeen times as many rods as there are cones in the human eye—about 120 million rods and 7 million cones in the retina of each eye. These rods and cones interconnect and converge to form networks of nerve fibers. About 1 million nerve fibers make up each optic nerve.

When the rods and cones receive light, they convert the light energy into nerve energy, which we will call a "visual impulse." This impulse travels out of the eye into the brain via the optic nerve at a speed of 423 miles per hour. It first reaches the middle of the brain, where a pair of "relay stations" combines the visual information being carried by the impulse with other sensory information. The impulse then travels to the very back part of the brain, the *visual cortex*. It is here that the brain interprets the shapes of objects and the spatial organization of scenes, and recognizes visual patterns as they belong to known objects–for example, it recognizes that a flower is a flower. Further visual process-ing is done at the sides of the brain, known as the *temporal lobes*. Once the brain has interpreted vital information about something the eyes have seen, it instantaneously transfers this information to the different areas of the brain that must play a part in the response. For example, if the information is that a car is moving toward you, this information is relayed to the *motor cortex*, which is the area that controls movement and enables you to get out of the car's way. The motor cortex is located in a band that goes over the top of your head, from just above one ear to just above the other ear.

Therefore, vision is really the combination of the eyeball receiving the light and the brain interpreting the signals from the eye and initi-ating a reaction. We will discuss this process of vision in more detail in the next chapter.

Refractive Errors

The process I have just described is how the normal eye and visual system function when working perfectly well. This condition of the eye being optically normal is called *emmetropia* (em-eh-TROH-pee-ah). (See Figure 1.2 on the facing page.) Not all eyes, unfortunately, are emme-tropic. Very often, something goes wrong and the visual process is dis-rupted. About 50 percent of adults in the United States have difficulty seeing clearly at distance, and about 60 percent have difficulty seeing up close with no corrective lenses. One of the more common problems

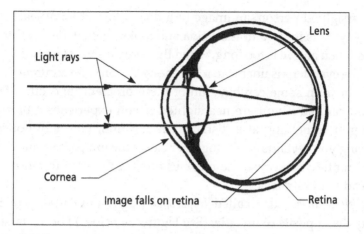

Figure 1.2. The Emmetropic Eye

is the mis-focusing of light as it is directed onto the retina. The light can focus too soon or too late, or it can be distorted. Because the bending of light is technically called "refraction," the mis-focusing of light in the eye is called a *refractive error.*

A refractive error can play a major role in the development of eyestrain. First, let's define the terms used to describe refractive errors. *Nearsightedness,* also called *myopia* (my-OH-pee-ah), means having good near vision but poor distance vision. (See Figure 1.3 below.) For

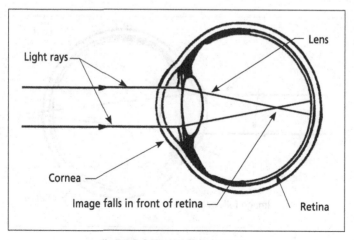

Figure 1.3. The Nearsighted Eye

the nearsighted person, an image of a distant object (of at least twenty feet away) falls in front of the retina and looks blurred. Nearsightedness results when an eye is too long, when the cornea is too steeply curved, or when the eye's lens is unable to relax enough to provide accurate distance vision, or from some combination of these problems and other factors.

You can tell if you are nearsighted if you experience a blur while looking at something at a distance. In addition, you may notice that squinting your eyelids closer together clears the image (to some degree). This squinting can cause the muscles around the eyes to tense, which will lead to eyestrain.

Farsightedness, also called *hyperopia* (high-per-OH-pee-ah), is not exactly the opposite of myopia. (See Figure 1.4 below.) For the farsighted person, the image of an object that is twenty feet or more away is directed past the retina, so that it looks blurred because it has not yet been brought into focus. Farsightedness occurs when the eye is too short or the cornea too flat, or from some combination of these and other factors. The main difference between nearsightedness and farsightedness is that the eye can increase its focal power by using its muscles to increase the shape of the crystalline lens, which can temporarily compensate for farsightedness, but it cannot reduce its power to compensate for nearsightedness.

As you might expect from the above situation, the muscles around and inside the eye become tense from overuse, thus creating a "strain" around the eyes. This is one of the more common reasons for eyestrain.

Theoretically, the surface of the cornea should be almost spherical in

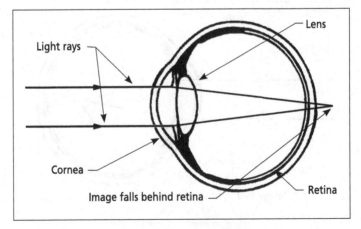

Figure 1.4. The Farsighted Eye

shape, like the surface of a ball, so that when light passes through it, it can be focused at a single point. Nature is not always perfect, however, and the cornea is often warped, resembling the side of a barrel, being flatter in one direction and steeper in the other direction. The lens, too, can be irregular in shape. These distortions can be significant enough so that the light that passes through the cornea and lens in the vertical orientation will focus at a different spot from the light that passes through in the horizontal orientation. Now you have two points of focus with a blur between them. This is known as *astigmatism* (ah-STIG-mah-tism). (See Figure 1.5 below.)

If the difference between these two points of focus is great enough, the eye will strain trying to decide which point of focus it should use. You might then develop occasional blurring of vision, tiring of the eyes, or possibly headaches, which all can be interpreted as eyestrain. Astigmatism in small amounts is very common and not of great concern. About 23 million Americans, however, have a significant amount of astigmatism, requiring correction. This is a major cause of eyestrain, but if a person with significant astigmatism has never seen clearly (having had the condition from birth), then the brain will adapt to fool the person into thinking they can see clearly. Glasses and contact lenses correct astigmatism because the curvature of the lens compensates for the curvature of the eye. This is a simple optical correction. Glasses or contacts, however, will not change the amount of astigmatism—that is, they will not cure the problem.

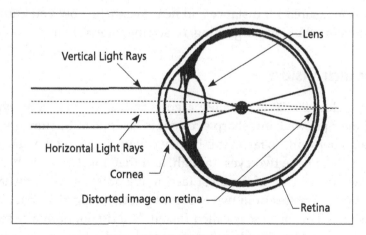

Figure 1.5. The Astigmatic Eye

Seeing Clearly Now

Think about the last time you visited your eye doctor's office. You probably got a full examination, had what seemed like a hundred different tests, and asked, "How are my eyes?" Your doctor may have said, "You have twenty-twenty vision!" Perhaps then you walked out of the office satisfied that your eyes were in good shape. Were they, though? What does "twenty-twenty," written as "20/20" for short, mean exactly?

The term *20/20 vision* is a notation that relates to the resolving power of the eye. An eye's resolving power is its sharpness of sight, which we can define as the ability to distinguish two points from each other and not see them as just one point. This resolution occurs at its maximum in the fovea portion of the retina. If your vision is 20/20, it means you're seeing at twenty feet what the "optically normal" eye can see at twenty feet—that is, that your eyes can distinguish one point from another on a specific line of characters from a standard eye chart placed twenty feet away. The standard chart, named Snellen chart (after Hermann Snellen, a Dutch ophthalmologist who introduced the chart to study visual acuity in 1862), is still the standard in eyesight testing. If your vision is, let's say, 20/40, it means that you can see at twenty feet what the normal eye can see at forty feet. You have to be closer to the object than normal. If your vision is 20/100, you must be at twenty feet while the normal eye can be one hundred feet away and see the same thing as clearly.

In short, the larger the bottom number is, the poorer the resolving power of your eye, which is also known as your visual acuity. Visual acuity is measured for distance and near vision. So now you know that 20/20 is something like a grading, or scaling, of eyesight.

Binocular Vision

Seeing a clear 20/20 is certainly a good indication that your eyes are doing their job well, but sharp eyesight is just one of the functions that your eyes perform. So far, in this book we have discussed the function of "the eye." We have two eyes, though, and they must work in harmony with each other. One of the most fascinating abilities of the visual system is to take images from two eyes and put them together to make just one picture. This process is called fusion. You do not normally see two images, so the idea might sound strange, but double vision can occur and is one of the most dangerous manifestations of vision problems leading to eyestrain. Imagine trying to hammer a nail and seeing two nails instead of one!

Here is how the brain puts two images into one picture. Let us assume that you have two eyes and they are both working about equally well. As you look at an object, each eye receives an individual image of that object. Both of these images are transmitted back to your brain, where they are then "fused" together into one image. In order for that to happen, however, both eyes must be pointed at the same object, at the same spot, with the images approximately equal in size and clarity. This is why the process is termed binocular vision.

Now, if one eye does not aim at the same spot as the other, each eye will see a slightly different view of the object, and the two images will not match up. When these images are transmitted back to your brain, they will stimulate two different groups of brain cells and you will experience two pictures, otherwise known as *diplopia* (dih-PLO-pee-ah), or double vision. After a short time, your brain will decide to suppress, or turn off, the image from the eye that is pointed in the wrong direction so that you can see one picture again, thus reducing the "strain" of two competing images. This suppression is necessary for our visual survival, but it is not the way we should use our visual system.

Suppression of an image is the brain's way of making our daily tasks easy and comfortable in stressful situations. Thus, while you might think that suppression of an image is devastating, it actually works pretty well. What is more serious, however, is when there is a competition between the eyes, when the eyes struggle to work together. It is competition that causes the person to grapple with reading tasks, and that can lead to poor reading comprehension, job performance, and, of course, eyestrain.

CONCLUSION

Our visual system is amazing and has evolved over the centuries to adapt to our daily viewing conditions. Eyestrain can arise when we try to use our eyes in new and unusual situations that are unnatural for us. It comes in many forms and with varied symptoms. We will now start to review how our eyes work in various daily tasks and how they can be strained if not prepared to do the job for which they were designed.

2

What Is Eyestrain and How Do You Know if You Have It?

One of the most common complaints heard in most eyecare practitioners' offices centers around persistent eyestrain. Eyestrain can lead to headaches, eye soreness, blurred vision, and many other issues that can interfere with clear, comfortable vision. In this chapter, we will review how eyestrain is defined and the causes of the condition.

TAKING A LOOK BACK

The current version of the species of man, *Homo sapiens,* first appeared between 300,000 and 400,000 years ago. Our ancestors were designed to survive in a difficult and challenging environment. Finding food, shelter, and protection were the first priorities, while the "comforts" of clothing and amenities were secondary. Their bodies developed to support their needs: flexibility, agility, and strength. If successful, they lived to the ripe old age of between twenty-five and thirty years old, according to most authorities.

Likewise, the eyes of our ancestors were designed for similar types of survival. They were situated in a frontal position so the visual fields could overlap and work together, creating the sense of stereoscopic vision—the ability to perceive depth. They are near the top of the body so as to afford the longest range of seeing. Since they were formed for mostly daytime viewing, our "bright" vision was keen; our night vision was adequate but secondary. The eyes were also developed so they could rotate and move in many directions, in conjunction with head movements, to be able to view a wide radius of the horizon. This design allowed a freedom of movement of the eyes so that they could see more easily without being strained.

This hunter-gatherer type of visual system is the same one we use today. We now, however, view our world for about sixteen hours a day, much of the time in artificial light and in an environment that is mostly within arm's reach. We read small items of text in various lighting situations for hours on end and struggle to meet deadlines. During much of the year, our eyes are exposed to very little daylight for an extended time. We are asking our eyes and visual system to adapt to these adverse conditions and they must make the necessary adaptations to assure our "survival." These changes are slow to develop and not always successful for what we need to accomplish. Oftentimes sacrifices are made in one area of vision for the sake of seeing better in other situations.

WHAT IS EYESTRAIN?

While eyestrain sounds like a simple concept, it is not that easily defined. The medical term for eyestrain is the condition known as *asthenopia*, (as-then-OH-pee-ah), which comes from the Greek words "asthenes," meaning weak, and "opia," meaning eye or vision. In fact, the actual definition from the *Dictionary of Visual Science* has several different variations of the condition, mostly related to from where the "strain" originates.

The general definition for asthenopia describes it as "a marked tendency for visual recognition to fade rapidly." (Of course, no eye-care practitioner is going to hear that coming from a patient who feels affected by eyestrain.) The *Dictionary of Visual Science* goes further when it attempts to define eyestrain. Its single definition is: "Asthenopia; ophthalmocopia; fatigue of the *ciliary muscle* or of some of the extrinsic (meaning external) muscles of the eyeball, due to errors of refraction or to imbalance of the ocular muscles; the symptoms are, in different cases, pain in the eyes, lacrimation (tearing), sties, headache, vertigo, nausea, and various other reflex symptoms."

The following conditions are forms asthenopia.

Accommodative Asthenopia

This term refers to eyestrain that is due to errors of refraction and the consequent strain on the ciliary muscle, which controls the focusing of the lens inside the eye.

Muscular Asthenopia

This term refers to eyestrain that is due to an imbalance of the extrinsic ocular muscles. These muscles attach to the outside of the eyeball and control eye movement. As you will recall from Chapter 1, the eyes must be pointing at the same object at the same time (eye coordination). If there is a tendency for the eyes to turn in too much, then they will strain to maintain a lock on the object being viewed. Conversely, the eyes may not turn in enough, and they may have to strain to try to maintain their aim at an object. Either situation is an ideal circumstance for muscular eyestrain.

Nervous Asthenopia

This term refers to eyestrain that is due to a functional or organic nervous disease. Any neurological disease can affect the comfort around eye movements. Many diseases, whether they are eye-related illnesses or occur in other parts of the body, can affect eye function. Since there are several nerves in and around the eyes, any disorder that affects nerves can make seeing more difficult and lead to eyestrain.

Tarsal Asthenopia

This term refers to eyestrain that is due to abnormal pressure of the eyelids on the globe of the eye. This is a rare occurrence, but if a medical condition presents with swelling of the eyelids, excessive pressure can cause discomfort. This is not so much related to the sagging of the eyelids that can accompany aging but rather a disorder of the glands within the eyelids, which can cause them to become stagnant and swell up.

Glare-Induced Asthenopia

This is a term I have decided to include in this section because modern computer use has created a reality in which people spend many hours looking at near images through glass. This circumstance can create excessive glare and light scatter, making images more difficult to see. This problem can also occur during night driving, when lights are scattered either through the windshield or due to a clouding of the structures within the eye (as often happens with cataract formation).

Digital Eyestrain

This term was coined in the early 1990s in response to the myriad of symptoms that people were experiencing while viewing computer screens. The original screens were designed like the original televisions (using a cathode ray tube projected onto a glass surface) and producing letters that were either white (on a black screen) or amber in color in a dot matrix pattern, which refers to a two-dimensional pattern of dots that is used to display images. This condition made it difficult to focus on letters, thus leading to eyestrain. (See Chapter 3 on page 19.)

Symptoms

From a patient's perspective, eyestrain can make itself known through a number of symptoms, including tired eyes, headaches, heavy eyes, blurred vision, fluctuating vision, "pulling" of the eyes (a feeling like the eye muscles are being "stretched"), visual hallucinations, double vision, and many more (we doctors have heard them all!). In general, however, eyestrain refers to any discomfort in or around the eyes that makes seeing difficult or blurred.

Here is another way to figure out if you have eyestrain: Go to a 3D movie! If you can enjoy the movie and perceive the true depth and action scenes of the movie with no problems, then your eyes are likely coordinated. If you notice that your vision is not clear, feel dizzy or possibly nauseated, get a headache, become light-headed, or experience any other physical symptoms, then you may have a binocular vision problem that can lead to eyestrain.

EYESTRAIN SYMPTOM CHECKLIST

The table on the following page is a checklist of symptoms that could lead to eyestrain along with their common causes, which you may be able to address. I hope you become aware enough of these causes to the point of avoiding the conditions that can strain your eyes.

Table 2.1. Symptom Checklist	
Symptom	**Possible Causes**
Headache (front of head)	Poor room lighting, poor contrast of letters on screen, squinting, convergence insufficiency, farsightedness, presbyopia
Headache (side or back of head)	Improper computer display position, poor contrast on screen, convergence insufficiency, farsightedness
Headache after school or work (difficulty with homework)	Poor focusing ability, convergence insufficiency, farsightedness
Headache (early in day)	Dietary imbalance, sleeping posture, unlikely eye-related
Distance vision blur	Myopia, accommodative insufficiency, inaccurate prescription glasses
Near vision blur	Farsighted, accommodative spasm, medicine interaction, poor multifocal lens placement
Dry eye	Nutritional imbalance, decreased blinking, dry environment
Watery eyes	Dry eye, pink eye, allergies, medicine interaction, viral infection
Red eyes	Pink eye, allergies
Difficulty night driving	Nearsightedness, cataract

As you can see, there are many causes of different symptoms of eyestrain. This fact makes an eye doctor's job more challenging. If you can troubleshoot some of these conditions on your own and then discuss your findings with your doctor, then your problem will most likely be able to be resolved appropriately and efficiently.

CONCLUSION

If you use your eyes for long periods to look at objects that are close to you, you'll likely experience some level of eyestrain. As described, our eyes are designed to look at a far distance during daylight hours with occasional near viewing. Our modern society, however, dictates that we use our eyes for close work more frequently, and this has become more intense since we became an "information society" dependent on computers and other electronics. In the next chapter, we will review the new demands on our visual system when looking at electrically generated digital display images.

3

Eyestrain in the Digital Age

The computer has been called "the machine that changed the world," and that is an accurate description. While computers have not completely replaced paper as a means of communication, they do allow us to work, shop, communicate, and play all from our desktops.

With this increase in digital technology, many individuals now suffer from numerous forms of physical discomfort after screen use. Some of these issues include carpal tunnel syndrome (wrist pain), back and neck aches, shoulder soreness, and other physical maladies. By far the most commonly noticed discomfort associated with computer use, however, has to do with the eyes. The American Optometric Association coined the term *computer vision syndrome* as those near-point viewing symptoms that can occur either during or after using a computer. Since the computer—or more accurately the digital viewing screen—has migrated from desktop to laptop to tablet to wrist (and even eyeglass lenses), the condition is now typically called digital eyestrain.

The Vision Council has studied this issue extensively and reports that about 90 percent of American adults report using digital devices for more than two hours a day, with almost 67 percent using two or more devices simultaneously. Of that 90 percent, 62 percent report experiencing symptoms of digital eyestrain. In connection with digital eyestrain, most people report experiencing the following symptoms:

- 32.4 percent report experiencing eyestrain
- 27.2 percent report experiencing dry eye

- 27.7 percent report experiencing headaches

- 27.9 percent report experiencing blurred vision

- 35 percent report experiencing neck and shoulder pain

Moreover, almost 80 percent report using digital devices, including TV, during the hour before going to sleep, and almost half of them report viewing again within the first hour they wake up. While more than 70 percent of American adults report their children receive more than two hours of screen time every day, nearly 25 percent are still not concerned about the impact of digital devices on their children's developing eyes. Recent surveys also show that the average teenager spends over seven hours a day viewing a digital image. Given that many school systems have transitioned to laptop and other digital display technologies for their lessons, these numbers are sure to rise. (See the inset "Digital Eyestrain in a Pandemic" on page 34.)

EYESTRAIN THROUGH THE AGES

The eyes are not fully formed structures at birth. While a baby's cornea is the same size as an adult's (which is why babies appear to have such large eyes), the remainder of the eyeball has yet to develop completely. The retina is mostly intact and formed, but the macula (central vision) is not yet attuned to seeing clearly. This process develops quickly over the first few months of life as the baby sees different objects and colors that stimulate the retina to mature properly.

Additionally, the aging process wreaks havoc on the various structures in the eye, so that older adults suffer either loss of clarity or degeneration of the tissue. The retina contains some of the most highly metabolic cells in the body, which means that they require a lot of energy in order to function properly. The use of computer displays is a relatively new task for humans, so there are still many unanswered questions as to what this usage can do to the eyes over a lifetime. Let us review the challenges that people may encounter at various age groups.

Young Children

The time from birth through the teenage years is typically known as the formative years. This is because children's bodies and minds are still in the growth stage. While the eye structure is well formed prior to the age of eight years old, the area of visual perception is still in an active developmental stage.

Television viewing takes up many of the idle hours of young children. The movement of images and funny characters draw the child to the screen for many hours a day. It is important to keep the youngsters viewing time limited and seated at a reasonable distance away from the screen for a few reasons. First, the farther away they are, the less they will have to accommodate, or focus, their eyes. Secondly, many times they will sit on the floor and crane their necks to see the screen. This can cause early-age neck and shoulder problems.

Additionally, two-dimensional images do not encourage the use of both eyes to coordinate themselves so that adequate *stereoscopic vision* (depth perception) develops. In addition, hand-eye coordination develops as youngsters learn to manipulate objects in their hands, which is absent in screen viewing.

Young Adults

Young adults in their late teens and twenties are typically multitaskers. They can switch back and forth between cell phone to laptop to tablet and connect with others on social media sites for hours at a time. Many teens opt to use several devices at a time. Once the social media time is over, they can spend more unlimited hours playing video games. While there may be some benefits associated with some of these games, they can also lead to physical maladies in the hands, neck, shoulders, and, of course, eyes.

Surveys show that over 90 percent of young adults check their cell phones approximately 262 times a day, with a number of those checks occurring within an hour of going to sleep. This dose of blue light can trick the brain into thinking it is getting ready for more activity rather than preparing to sleep. If your teen has difficulty falling or staying asleep, this is one area to consider.

As mentioned, these days many schools are switching over to display-based technologies in the classroom as well. Most classrooms were designed to accommodate paper-based tasks and lighting that supports such tasks. Computer displays, however, require different light levels. Hopefully, schools will retrofit their lights to accommodate digital displays.

Thirty-Somethings

Adults in their thirties spend a good percentage of their time in the workplace, oftentimes in cubicles. You might think that the workplace has all the accommodations to make computer display viewing an acceptable task, but this is not always the case. Thin budgets and lack of knowledge of basic ergonomic principals can lead to employees who struggle at their desks. *Ergonomics* is the study of people in their work environments, which is performed in an effort to prevent injury or discomfort due to the makeup of their work environments. It covers all areas of computer work (the work environment and tasks performed in this area). The area of study of visual ergonomics deals with the eyestrain that computer-display users experience during or after display viewing. We will review some of these concerns later in this chapter.

Moreover, when they are not at work, many spend their leisure hours playing video games. At this age, some of these "gamers" might consider a career in video game tournaments. Most people would be surprised that the average age of a video game player is 37 years old! This area, known as e-sports, is a huge industry, and competitions draw thousands of spectators. These "e-athletes" spend hours upon hours viewing computer displays, oftentimes without much blinking to refresh their eyes. This staring habit is a sure-fire cause of eyestrain—one of the most common complaints of this group.

Forty-Somethings

As adults in their forties experience vision changes associated with a loss of focusing ability, many face challenges trying to maintain a clear image while looking at a near distance. While this is a gradual process, which begins after the age of ten, it becomes noticeable in the early forties because this loss of clarity reaches the typical reading distance (about sixteen inches). Surveys show that about 66 percent of these folks experience symptoms of digital eyestrain.

Computer use continues to grow in this group because of the growing popularity of online shopping, keeping track of professional sports, following finances, and other daily endeavors.

Fifty-Somethings

This category of display viewer was the original early adopters of digital technology, having used computers in the 1990s. Thus, most of these people depend on computers and laptops to do a myriad of tasks. Over 65 percent of this group exhibits signs of digital eyestrain, having already stared at screens for more than three hours a day for up to fifteen years, with some spending more than five hours a day viewing digital screens.

Sixties and Over

Adults aged sixty and over represent the fastest growing group of Internet users because of their interest in health-related topics. This population has been quick to monitor their health via data captured through wearable devices. They have also been eager to adopt technologies that support active living. More than half of these aging eyes, however, experience symptoms of digital eyestrain, spending upward of five hours or more viewing screens each day.

This group is most likely to use a computer or laptop for tasks such as getting directions, finding a recipe, doing research, checking social media, and playing games.

THREE ASPECTS OF DIGITAL EYESTRAIN

There are three aspects of display viewing to consider where eyestrain is involved:

1. What are your work habits?

2. What is your work environment?

3. What is your vision status?

Let us look at these three areas of concern to see how to prevent, or at least reduce, the likelihood of eyestrain.

Work Habits

Digital displays have been adapted to many different work situations, so arranging the display on a desk will depend on how often the worker must look at the screen. There are several options for differing jobs. For example, workers in customer support, who have a headset and view the screen only for extended periods, must remember to take more breaks from this constant viewing distance. On the other hand, someone who performs data entry will likely be viewing the hard copy, with occasional viewing of the display screen. If computer users perform word processing, they will likely be going back and forth between hard copy and the display screen. Here it is important to remember that the two sources should be in close proximity to each other in order to avoid excessive eye and head movements. Lighting for each source, however, might pose a problem, which we will discuss later in this chapter.

An extreme example of digital eyestrain would be a computer programmer who will be "locked in" to viewing the screen for extended hours at a time. Given that a programmer's income is dependent on getting the work done on a deadline, this can mean spending up to eighteen hours a day viewing a display screen. (Yes; I had a patient state this number as fact.)

The "Three B" Approach

In the face of so much digital viewing, I recommend a system known as the "three B" approach to balance the situation. This approach states, "Blink, breathe, and break." It is very important to blink to avoid dry eye disease and to maintain a uniform tear layer on the surfaces of the eyes. Blinking allows nutrients to feed the cornea properly and creates an even layer of tears to focus the light into the eye with clarity. Breathing in stressful situations (like deadlines) can become shallow and inefficient, thus reducing blood flow to the head, resulting in tired eyes and eyestrain.

When it comes to taking breaks, I created the "20-20-20" rule. This recommendation is to take a 20-second break, every 20 minutes, during which you would look 20 feet away. Doing so will allow you to unfocus your eyes and relax the focusing muscles. Now, this 20-20-20 rule will not assure that your eyesight does not deteriorate or reverse nearsightedness, but it will reduce your level of eyestrain. I developed this rule because of studies that showed that shorter and more frequent breaks were more effective at reducing strain for computer users. so that people would easily remember the rule when thinking about their eyes.

Work Environment

The workplace of the 1950s, in which typewriters sat upon desktops, has been replaced by the modern workplace, which is filled with cubicles, each with a tiny space occupied by a computer display. In the early 1980s and up until the late 1990s, most of these displays were variations of the television technology that once used a cathode ray tube, or CRT, to display pictures. This technology created an image using a "gun" that shot electrons onto a phosphorescent screen in a vacuum. This is where the images of letters were formed in a dot-like pattern. These monitors took up quite a bit of desk space, so their screens were typically close to the workers, thus requiring more focusing effort. In addition, the glass that covered the screen was highly reflective, so reflections typically interfered with viewing the screen. Eyestrain was a common complaint with these screens.

The introduction of the flat display screen marked a big change in technology and soon became the standard for desktop computers. This type of screen uses liquid crystal display, or LCD, technology, and comes with many advantages (clearer letter configuration, thinner profile, larger screen, etc.), so it quickly took over. Workers could now fit multiple screens on the same workspace, and they could see their images much clearer. There were still some drawbacks, though, such as inconsistent colors, decreased contrast, a fixed resolution (no changes in text size), and more.

Nevertheless, despite these initial problems, LCD technology thrived, and it continues to be the default in digital displays. It has improved and addressed many of its problems, of course, but eyestrain is still an issue for many computer users.

With the advent of tablet displays came the light-emitting diode, or LED. This technology was developed in the 1960s and eventually progressed enough to be incorporated into computer displays. The light distribution for the LED lights was very high in the blue light range of the visible spectrum, where blue light is the highest energy of light reaching the retina. There is quite a bit of controversy over blue light and computer displays, in fact, but most experts realize that the amount of blue light coming from a computer display is minimal compared with the blue light from the sun.

Another significant factor in eyestrain is lighting. Paper use depends on light reflecting off the paper into the eyes, whereas display technology has its own light, sourced from behind the screen. Thus, if someone is using both paper and digital displays in the same office, there is likely going to be one or the other that is not properly lit for comfortable viewing.

To address this lighting issue, you need to follow your parents' sage advice: Don't watch TV in the dark. It is true that a screen will appear brighter if a room is completely dark (as it often is for air traffic controllers, for example). The retina, however, does not like high-contrast lighting environments for extended viewing. It is a significant cause of eyestrain. It is best if the background of a display screen and its immediate surroundings' illumination are approximately equal.

Glare is another type of lighting issue that is common with viewing computer displays. There are two types of glare: discomfort and disability, and both can lead to eyestrain. Discomfort glare causes one to look away from a bright light source. Disability glare impairs the vision of objects without necessarily causing discomfort. This type of glare is often caused by the reflection of light within the eyeball, reducing the contrast between task and glare source so that the task cannot be distinguished. When glare is so intense that vision is completely impaired, it is called "dazzle." Most examples of glare are the discomfort type, and while not as intense as disability glare, this type can cause eyestrain and diminish work efficiency.

There are several ways to address glare in the office. Here are a few options:

- **Turn off the offending light.** If there is a light source shining directly into your eyes, it will likely be the source of the eyestrain. Many light fixtures in the workplace are "double-switched," having one switch turn on two of the bulbs while a second switch turns on the other two in the fixture. Turning on only one switch will reduce the overall lighting in the workplace by half.

- **Rotate your workstation.** Make sure that uncovered windows are off to the sides, not behind your screen or behind you.

- **Draw the curtains or blinds.** Curtains or blinds won't help if they aren't closed! Remember that outdoor light is not reliable and changes throughout the day, so uncovered windows are not the best options for viewing computer displays.

- **Avoid bright reflective surfaces.** White desktops or white clothing can actually reflect light back onto some screens and decrease the contrast of an image.

- **Use task lights.** Task lights are directional and so should be directed toward hard copy and away from a display screen.

- **Adjust screen brightness.** Remember that a display has two major adjustments: brightness and contrast. Adjust each until you find comfortable settings.

- **Use a visor.** While sitting at your screen, use your hand as a visor on your forehead. If your eyes then feel more comfortable and their muscles relax, then your lighting is a problem. Using a visor at your workstation can help solve this source of eyestrain.

Vision Status

There are many types of eye problems that can contribute to eyestrain. Let's take a look at some of the more common ones to see how they can cause unwanted issues.

Farsightedness

When you are farsighted, you must use the focusing ability of the crystalline lens just about every minute of the day. Even when looking at a distant object, the eyes must actively focus to bring the image to the appropriate point on the retina. This requires the ciliary muscle (which surrounds the lens) to flex, therefore increasing focal power. The ciliary muscle is meant to be flexed, of course, but it can become overstimulated. Such overstimulation can create a strain when a person is trying to see clearly for extended periods.

To make matters worse, a farsighted eye not only has to do extra focusing on distant objects but also needs to do additional focusing when looking closer than twenty feet. This excess focusing is a guaranteed way to experience eyestrain.

Nearsightedness

While nearsighted eyes have difficulty seeing clearly at a distance, they will often strain to see more clearly. This circumstance most often occurs when a person squints, squeezing their eyelids close together. This movement actually helps to some degree, as it narrows the peripheral light rays that create a blurred image on the retina, allowing the central rays to focus on the macula. Most nearsighted people, though, cannot squint hard enough for long enough to clear the image appropriately. Their eyelid muscles become strained with excessive use.

Astigmatism

You may recall that astigmatism is an optical distortion that creates a spread-out image near the retina so that vision blurs when looking both far and near. Because there is no "point" of light for the eye to focus on, the ciliary muscle continually contracts and relaxes, trying to find the best clear point for proper vision. Since it never finds a clear point, it will often tire and allow just a blurred image to form on the retina. This is one of the more common causes of eyestrain.

Binocular Imbalance

We must keep in mind that we have two eyes to use for all of our viewing scenarios. The two images generated in the two eyes travel along the optic nerves to the brain and eventually reach the back part of the brain, which processes the images. If the two images are not very close to identical, however, the brain will have difficulty fusing them into one image, causing a person to see double, or the brain may tune out one of the images. Prior to getting to this point, the eyes can struggle to align properly, and this is where eyestrain takes hold. The eyes should not have to fight one another to be properly aligned, but if they are not coordinated properly, fight they will. The good news is that this coordination process can be trained with a series of techniques through a program of vision therapy. (See Resources on page 167.)

Dry Eye

Studies confirm that computer users blink about one-third as often as those reading text on paper. Thus, it is not surprising that they complain of dry eye much more often. *Dry eye disease* can cause the tear film to thin and interestingly it also causes reflex tearing, which will thicken the tears. Both of these conditions can lead to eyestrain.

Additionally, most desktop computer displays are viewed so that the top of the display is above eye level. This requires the user to look straight ahead when viewing the display. Unfortunately, this is not how our eyes work. In fact, when our eyes converge their line-of-sight to look up close, they automatically look lower in the visual field. This is why it is more comfortable to read text in a lower line-of-sight, as with books on a desk. Therefore, lowering the display screen so that the top of the display is at eye level, will allow you to view the text on the display in a lower posture, allowing an easier blink rate. Also, be sure to tilt the screen back at the top so that your line-of-sight is perpendicular to the plane of the screen.

This is also where my "20-20-20" rule comes into play. By giving yourself more short breaks during the day, you allow your eyes to relax and blink more often, thus reducing eyestrain.

Cataracts

A *cataract* is a degeneration of the crystalline lens within the eye. This degeneration causes the lens to lose its clarity, becoming "foggy." Some believe that this is a normal progression of the aging process, which is understandable since 90 percent of cataract patients are over the age of sixty.

When computers were first used in the workplace, there was a fear of the display emitting radiation that might cause a cataract. Surveys showed, however, that just the older people reported this type of visual distortion, so it was likely more that aging was the determining factor.

Unfortunately, there is no cure for a cataract. Given that the lens receives most of its nutrients in the eye from the aqueous humor, which has twenty-six times more vitamin C in it than any other fluid in the body, it makes sense that antioxidants might help at least delay cataract formation. On a more positive note, it is the most common surgery performed in the United States. The procedure removes the degenerated lens and replaces it with an artificial lens, which will remain clear throughout the remainder of the patient's lifetime.

Other Medical Conditions

We must remember that the eyes are an integral part of the body, so things that affect our bodies can affect our eyes. Where computer display viewing is concerned, it is common for neck and back problems to be associated with these tasks. We know that the "eyes lead the body," such that if the eyes are strained, then the body will try to adjust to reduce that stress. This is why neck and backaches are associated with not only computer use but also eyestrain in general. Once the eyes are clear and comfortable, then the rest of the body can follow suit.

When it comes to kids, of course, this solution is not so easily accomplished. Kids do not realize how much time has passed when they are engrossed in a video game or texting with friends. A study from Canada's McMaster University found that kids with video game addictions sleep less, which in turn elevates blood pressure, lowers good cholesterol (HDL), and raises triglycerides, in addition to narrowing the arteries in the retina. We need to put limits on kids' use of video displays so they can develop physically as well as mentally.

DISPLAY TECHNOLOGIES

Each form of digital display technology has its unique attributes. Some are very large displays (e.g., desktop displays), while some can be worn on your wrist (e.g., smart watches). We will review each of these devices to see how eyestrain might develop in association with their use, and to learn how to adjust these displays to reduce the strain on our eyes.

Desktop Monitors

The first computer display was the desktop monitor that was a component of the computer system, which comprised a central processing unit (CPU), a keyboard, and a CRT display. These three items were to take the place of the workplace typewriter, however they took up more room than the typewriter did. The solution was to go vertical with the display unit, putting it on top of the CPU (for desktop units), assuming that this would be a proper location to best view the display.

There were several problems with this design, but the main visual challenge was that people were now looking in a more straight-ahead posture with their eyes instead of the downward gaze used on typewriters. The poorly configured images (the "dot-matrix" design of letters), the glare off the shiny glass screen, the room lighting glare into the eyes, and the higher than normal viewing angle all led to eyestrain issues.

Today we have flat-screen displays on our desktops (and very often more than just one display for each computer). These screens use a different technology to generate the images on the display and are much more refined than CRT technology. The positive aspects of a flat screen are several: a) they are thinner, so they can be relocated on the desktop to best adjust to the user; b) the images are closer to print clarity; c) they are larger, so more data can be seen on the screen at one time; and d) they use less power than the CRTs. There is still some glare off the front of the screen, though. While more diffuse, it can cause discomfort glare and degrade the image to create more eyestrain.

Laptop Monitors

Laptop computers (also called notebooks) have made computing more mobile. Flat-screen technology, being thin and light, allows the screen to be positioned in any orientation. Given that the keyboard and the screen are attached to each other, a laptop display tends to be positioned closer to the user than a desktop display. As with all near-point objects, the closer to the eyes they are, the more the eyes must focus to clear the image. Without proper eye focusing ability, eyestrain will occur.

Tablets

Tablet displays (iPads, etc.) have eliminated the need for keyboards, instead using virtual keyboards generated on their screens. The quality of a tablet display has improved to such a degree that one would think eyestrain would not be associated with this device. Most tablets do not have any type of support structure, however, so they require an after-market solution to keep the user from holding the screen for extended periods. These supports can allow the display to be held in almost any position, with or without using your hands. Thus, they can also be positioned in a poor configuration for optimum viewing. If not placed appropriately, eyestrain is sure to be a side effect of using a tablet.

Cell Phones

With the advent of even smaller displays, we now use cellular telephones, or cell phones, for almost all of our daily activities. Our phones have become address books, maps, magnifiers, flashlights, cameras, communication devices, and more. Cell phone screen technology is excellent, so we cannot truly say that the screen is a major cause of eye problems and eyestrain. Nevertheless, the fact is that we use cell phones for just about everything, and are in the habit of looking at them for endless hours on a daily basis. This constant viewing surely leads to excessive eyestrain, no matter the quality of a cell phone's screen.

Studies show that people check their phones over two hundred times a day on average. While this device is our main connection to the wider world, that statistic does seem troubling. The best option here is to limit the amount of time looking at your cell phone. Although content providers are more than happy for you to watch their products on your cell phone, these devices were never intended to be screens on which to watch full-length movies, etc. Short spurts of viewing should be fine, though.

Video Games

The video game industry has exploded with millions of gamers and it is getting bigger all the time. Vision while playing a video game differs significantly from routine TV viewing. First, the images are moving much faster and the details are more refined in a video game. The monitor tends to be closer to the user and the tasks involved often require acute hand-eye coordination. The eye movements associated with playing video games, which include tracking and scanning, can easily induce eyestrain in the untrained user. There are actually some video games that have been designed to improve the eye movements of the user, but they are meant to be played under the supervision of an eyecare professional in a vision-training environment. To reduce strain on the eyes, a complete eye examination, including an evaluation of eye-movement abilities, should be an annual event.

Television

As previously mentioned, TV viewing significantly differs from viewing a computer display. First, most TVs are placed farther away than displays, and thus require less focusing effort. Moreover, most TV viewing does not require reading of small detailed letters and words; it is more involved with following moving pictures. Additionally, most TV viewing is done while sitting on a soft, cushioned surface (like a sofa), which affords the viewer a more reclined position. This position creates an effective lowering of the viewing angle and less opening of the eyelids, allowing for less effort exerted when blinking.

One question that is often asked is, "How far should you sit from your TV?" One study explored the effect of TV size, illumination, and viewing angle on preferred viewing distance of high-definition liquid crystal display television. Results showed that the most often preferred viewing distance was about nine feet. The larger the TV size, the longer the preferred viewing distance was, at around three to four times the width of screen. In addition, the greater the illumination, the longer the preferred viewing distance was. The more off-center from the direct front view, the shorter the viewing distance seemed to be.

HOW TO CHOOSE A MONITOR

Choosing a computer monitor can be a daunting task. I liken the process to someone who goes into an electronics store to purchase a stereo system. The first question that is often asked is, "How much do you want to spend?" This assumes that the customer has excellent hearing and can discern subtle nuances in the sounds coming from different units. Thus, the first question should be, "How good is your hearing?"

Similarly, when choosing a computer display, you need to know how acute your vision is. If you have poor eyesight, purchasing a top-quality monitor will not be an efficient use of your funds. So, maybe an eye exam to test for computer-viewing distance would be warranted prior to reviewing computer displays.

Your choice of monitor depends on what you will mainly be using your computer for, and this question can be answered looking at three overarching categories: general/business use, professional visuals, and gaming. General/business use monitors can be found at home or work offices and are mostly used to run office applications, web browsers, and computer programs that do not need heavy graphics processing. As a result, you will usually be able to tell which monitors are for general use based on their low price tags. Because these products support frugal budgets, your computer will not need any high-end specs or up-to-date upgrades to utilize these standard monitors properly.

If you are a digital artist, content creator, or just looking to get started in the field of visual entertainment, being acquainted with what a professional design/editing monitor can offer is necessary. Whether you are designing something that will be displayed in print or on a website, getting the right colors (and thus creative ambiance) can easily be taken for granted. If you decide to cut costs and go for a lower-end monitor, the colors you may have had in mind when finishing a project could look quite different on other screens. Of course, you will need to have a machine that can run high-end graphics programs, such as Adobe Photoshop or Apple's Final Cut Pro.

Gaming monitors need to be fast. "Fast" in monitor terms refers to each display's refresh rate and response time. Fast refresh rates typically run at around 240Hz, which means that your game's imagery will be displayed at a range of 240 frames per second (that is very fast). Display response times can be crucial in determining whether a monitor's refresh rate looks good, since they are a measurement of how quickly colors can be shifted. Currently the fastest response time on a monitor is 1 millisecond (ms).

As their name implies, ultrawide monitors stretch out left and right to provide you with more screen space, which can simulate the productive efficiency of using two or three monitors at the same time. Great for displaying multiple applications at once, ultrawide monitors can be a professional's business display of choice.

Digital Eyestrain in a Pandemic

In the year 2020, the COVID-19 pandemic took hold and became an incredible challenge for our entire planet. Since the best option for reducing the effects of the virus was to isolate from one another, people had to put their lives on hold until things resolved. This reality meant almost no person-to-person interaction. The alternative was to use our display technologies and Internet capabilities to try to interact with people virtually.

Schools closed down in favor of online classes. Instead of having students in a classroom where they had various viewing distances (across the room or to their neighbors), kids were stuck looking at computer displays for about six hours a day. Interviews with students confirmed that their learning skills had deteriorated as a result. Many felt stressed and anxious.

Eyecare professionals also saw a rise in visual stress issues in their patients that were students. Many had become more nearsighted, and some now had binocular vision problems. Dry eye disease was appearing at younger ages, and focusing problems were being exacerbated. Fortunately, the use of properly prescribed reading glasses or computer glasses could make a huge difference. This fact illustrates just how important eye exams are, and how the use of proper eyewear can make an impact on this "new normal" we are all facing.

EYEWEAR TO ELIMINATE DIGITAL EYESTRAIN

Eyewear is available with lenses that feature magnification as well as anti-reflective and blue light-filtering capabilities to help reduce symptoms of digital eyestrain. (Contact lenses can also offer similar benefits.) You do not have to sacrifice style (or your bank account) for function when it comes to eyewear for eyestrain. These specialized lenses can be incorporated into virtually any pair of frames available at a variety of price points, so you can choose eyewear that complements your personal look and is within your budget, while also meeting your eye health needs. We will discuss more of these specifics in upcoming chapters.

The Vision Council recommends individuals and their children visit eyecare providers to discuss their digital habits and what solutions are available to relieve symptoms of digital eyestrain. Only 20.5 percent of people report having an annual eye exam and discussing their digital device usage with their eyecare providers, with about 30 percent reporting the same in connection with their children.

As you can now see, vision in the digital age can present many challenges for the eyes and visual system in general. In the next chapter, we will look at a visual task that has been with us for much longer than computer displays: reading on paper. Yes, people still read books printed on paper, and we are still a long way from having a paperless society. Now, if we can just get kids to figure out how to open a book . . .

4

Children and Eyestrain

Children are just as likely to be subject to eyestrain as adults are. For parents, the issue may be first identifying if their child has a problem. Young children just assume that their vision is the same as everyone else's. This is because they have no way to make any comparisons. They simply take it for granted that they are seeing what everyone else is seeing from the very beginning of their lives. Yet, as children grow, their eyes should normally develop along with the rest of their bodies during maturation. Except for severe eye disorders, the fact is that young children with subtle vision problems are not aware that they have any problems with their eyes. If they are unable to see the leaves on a tree from across the street or the letters on a blackboard from the rear of a classroom, they accept it as normal and say nothing.

Unfortunately, this is more of a common problem than most parents think. Studies show that one out of every twenty preschool children in the United States has a vision problem that can contribute to eyestrain. In addition, if uncorrected, it can lead worsening vision as well as a severe learning disability. Between 80 and 85 percent of our learning comes through vision. The good thing is that most vision problems are correctable if detected early. Therefore, as a parent, it is your job to talk with your child and find out what is happening with his or her vision. By your identifying a vision problem early, you can help your child alleviate the potential problems that come with poor eyesight.

One of the most unanswered questions by new parents is, "How old should a child be for their first eye examination?" Most parents think that their pediatrician covers this by having children read an eye chart across the room. While pediatricians are highly trained specialists, vision testing is rudimentary in their practices. Surprisingly, pediatric

37

optometrists like to see children who are one year old (or earlier if parents notice any irregularities). Routine exams can start at three years old and every year prior to the school term during grade school. School nurses perform minimal vision screenings at school, which will likely not pick out a vision-related reading condition. It is much easier to prevent a vision-based learning problem than to remedy one.

This chapter will show you some simple techniques for testing your child's vision, and for helping to improve his or her visual perception. It will also discuss some of the common signs to look for when trying to determine if your child has a vision issue. If you have any doubts about whether your child's vision is developing on schedule, or if you should detect a problem, I advise you to consult your developmental optometrist or pediatrician. Developmental optometrists have a special interest in visual development process and visual perception. (See Resources on page 167.)

SCHOOL PROVIDES THE FIRST CLUES

School and vision—the two are practically synonymous. School is for learning, and most of learning relies on vision. All the skills and abilities that children develop during the preschool years come into play during the remaining school years. Moreover, the most demanding test of visual abilities is reading, and more reading occurs in school than anywhere else.

Unfortunately, four out of ten grade-school children in the United States are visually handicapped for adequate school achievement. Visual handicaps include not only seeing a blurry image when looking at a blackboard, but also poor eye movement *(oculomotor coordination)*, crossed eyes (strabismus), lazy eye (amblyopia), focusing insufficiency, perceptual problems, and developmental delays.

WHAT SHOULD NORMAL VISION LOOK LIKE

Eye movements involved in the reading process are among the most complicated movements in the body. The muscles that control focusing and the muscles that control eye movement must work in perfect harmony for optimum reading comprehension. Let us look at a few of the important visual skills children need in school.

- *Near-vision acuity.* This is ability to see things fourteen to sixteen inches away (reading distance) clearly with both eyes. It should not be confused with nearsightedness, which implies that distance vision is blurry.

- *Distance-vision acuity.* This is the ability to see things at least twenty feet away with sharpness and very little effort. In addition, it is not to be confused with farsightedness, which implies that near vision is difficult.

- *Accommodation.* This is the ability of the eyes to adjust for near-point tasks easily. This process must be performed comfortably and must be maintained for long periods.

- *Focusing flexibility.* This is the ability to alternate between distance and near vision quickly and effortlessly.

- *Binocular coordination.* This is the ability of both eyes to work together as a team using either distance or near vision. Tiring, double vision, poor reading ability, and headache are a few signs of inadequate binocular coordination.

- *Adequate field of vision.* This is the ability to see up, down, left, and right while focusing on one spot. This saves unnecessary head and eye movements, and is crucial for reading.

The good news is that, if deficiencies are evident in these types of eye movements, the child can perform techniques to rectify the problem. Sometimes a simple program of eye movement sessions can retrain the eyes and visual system to perform with more accuracy, thus allowing better word recognition and perception. Please do not confuse these techniques with eye "exercises," which claim to strengthen eye muscles. In over 99 percent of cases, eye muscles are strong enough to move an eyeball; the problem lies in coordination between the eyes, which occurs in the brain. We will offer some of these simple tests at the end of this book. (See Chapter 11 on page 141.)

THE SIGNS OF EYE TROUBLE

Many times, eye problems show up as behavioral difficulties, as a result of which a child might be labeled as lacking attention, slow to learn, or disruptive. A child's difficult behavior may have an underlying learning disability such as dyslexia or attention deficit hyperactivity disorder (ADHD), but it is important to rule out a vision problem before assigning a label. The following signs and symptoms are the A-B-C-Ds that may signal vision trouble during the school-aged years.

[A]   Appearance of the Eyes

[B]   Behavior

[C]   Complaints

[D]   Disabilities in Learning

Appearance of the Eyes

By observing the state of your child's eyes, you can detect a variety of potential problems. Some signs are easy to spot, while others are subtle. Although you should not jump to conclusions, the subtle signs that appear repeatedly are worth a visit to an eyecare professional. There are five signs to watch for in your observations.

Crossed Eyes or Wandering Eye

It may not seem as obvious as you might expect, but misalignment of one of the eyes occurs in about 8 percent of the population. On the other hand, it is extremely rare for both eyes to be *crossed* or *walleyed*. You have to see with at least one eye, so one usually aims properly. The general medical term for the condition in which both eyes do not aim at the same point in space is *strabismus* (strah-BIZ-mas). If one eye turns in, it is termed *esotropia* (ee-so-TROH-pee-ah). If one eye is turns out, it is called *exotropia* (ex-oh-TROH-pee-ah). This is different from lazy eye, which is termed *amblyopia* (am-blee-OH-pee-ah).

If an eye has amblyopia, it is not correctable to 20/20 with any lens powers. It might, however, be pointing to the corresponding point as the other eye. It is often observed that one can have both amblyopia and strabismus together. The theory is that, if an eye is not pointing correctly, then it will not contribute to the vision perceived in the brain, and the eye will not develop to see clearly, that is, it will not be correctable to 20/20.

You can easily test for strabismus in your child. Have the child look at your fingertip about sixteen inches away with both eyes open. As you watch the right eye, cover the left eye with your hand. Did the right eye move when you did this? Now reverse the process. Watch the left eye and cover the right eye. There should be no movement of the eye you are watching when the other eye is covered. If there is, then that eye was not used to fixate on the target, and thus the eyes are not being used together.

Once again, it is important to remember that control of the eye muscles is not usually a muscle strength problem. It involves coordination between the two eyes, and this coordination occurs in the brain. It is due to this fact that therapy is available, which can resolve the condition. A program of vision therapy sets up visual conditions that guide the eyes to work in conjunction with each other.

A medical approach to treating crossed eyes is to rearrange the eye muscles that control eye movement surgically. The procedure shortens or relocates the muscle to improve the "aiming" of the eye. Unfortunately, it is not an exact science, and there is no way to gauge accurately how far to move the muscle, so over- or under-correction is possible. Carefully consider whether this is the best approach to aligning the eyes.

Red Eyes

The white of the eye is supposed to be mostly white. Some normal blood vessels, however, are typically visible on the surface. If there is excessive redness, it can be a sign of trouble, but it is not easy to determine what the cause of the problem might be. This warrants a visit to the eye doctor. If it is *pink eye*, which refers to an inflammation of the conjunctiva, it can be very contagious, so take precautions.

Watery Eyes

Overly wet eyes can be an indication of eyestrain, dry eye, or allergies, among a few other disorders. An eyecare professional will be able to check the various causes of this problem and make the proper recommendation.

Encrusted Lids

The eyelids have glands inside of them that produce an oily fluid to support the normal coating of the tears produced on the surface of the exposed eye. If there is crusting on the edges of the eyelids, it is likely a type of infection is present, which will likely be treatable by an eyecare professional.

Frequent Styes

A *stye* is an infection in the gland near the eyelash follicle. It can look similar to a *chalazion* (sha-LAY-zee-on), which is an infection of the glands within the eyelids. Either issue should be managed with a treatment of hot compresses applied several times a day. If it does not resolve in a week or so, then it might need medical treatment.

Behavior

The way your child behaves when looking at an object such as a page in a book or a computer screen can provide you with a clue if your child has an eye problem. There are a number of easy-to-spot signs that your child may have a visual impairment.

Squinting or Closing of One Eye

The two eyes are supposed to work together smoothly. If a child cannot easily do this, then it would be easier to close one eye to perform near viewing. Notice if your child leans on one hand while reading, as that hand could be covering one eye! This indicates that the two eyes are struggling to work together. If not addressed, this issue might lead to a misalignment of the eyes or lazy eye.

Rigid Body Posture

When sitting and reading for long periods, your child could have muscle spasms or cramps. Our bodies need to move regularly, and sitting can lead to poor circulation and rigid body postures. Since the eyes lead the body, this might indicate a struggle for the eyes to work efficiently.

Avoidance of Close Work

There are studies that show that about 90 percent of juvenile delinquents suffer from some sort of visual disability. It seems that, if they cannot pay attention to reading, they will just get into trouble doing other activities. Children should be able to sit and read for a reasonable amount of time without fidgeting or constantly getting up for snacks or TV breaks. Taking routine breaks from intense near viewing, of course, is preferred. As a guide, we recommend the "20-20-20" rule: Every 20 minutes, take 20 seconds, and look 20 feet away.

Rocking Back and Forth

This habit is a sure sign of stress. The rocking back and forth is a release of strain on the body. This action can make it more difficult for the eyes to follow the words on the page, inducing eyestrain.

Head Turning

Turning of the head while reading can indicate a few different problems. First, it suggests that one eye may be more dominant than the other, putting more strain on one eye. Secondly, it is stressful for the neck muscles to maintain an awkward posture, which can lead to a misalignment of the eyes and eyestrain.

Excessive Head Movement

The eyes are very mobile structures and have many muscles that control their movement. They should easily move independent of the head. Excessive head movement indicates that the eyes are not coordinating properly and can cause issues such as vertigo.

Sitting Too Close to the Work

The closer you sit to an object, the more focusing demand on the eyes. A convenient measure of a proper reading distance is to measure the distance from the middle knuckle to the elbow. This length is the optimum reading distance for a child.

Using a Finger to Read

While hand-eye coordination is important, at some point the eyes need to lead without assistance from the hands. If a child uses a finger to help aim the eyes, then it is a sign of immature eye movement. Eye movement exercises can help resolve this problem.

Blinking a Lot and with Effort

The eyes need to maintain their moisture and blinking is essential to meet this need. Too much (or not enough) blinking, however, shows either a poor wetting of the eye's surface or a struggle to clear the image. Either way, effortful blinking is a sure way to get tired and strained eyes.

Rubbing the Eyes during or after Short Periods of Reading

There are many reasons for rubbing the eyes, but drying of the eyes is a leading cause. One must rule out allergic reaction or bacterial infection that might cause this condition.

Complaints

Some of these common signs are either harder to detect or not necessarily seen as vision issues.

Blurred Vision

One of the first signs that can let a parent know that there might be a vision problem in a child is blurred vision. As we noted earlier, however, many children may not realize that their vision is not as sharp as their friends' or other people's vision. They many just accept blurred vision as their normal visual ability. Nevertheless, when reading, a child should be able to see the letters and words clearly; they should never appear blurred. This type of image can easily spark eyestrain.

Burning or Itchy Eyes

These complains usually follow the rubbing of the eyes after short periods of reading. Pink eye and allergies are common causes of these symptoms but also indicators of dry eye.

Double Vision

Seeing double is a sure sign of loss of coordination between the two eyes. In older adults, it can be a significant sign of nerve disease (for example, multiple sclerosis), but in younger children, poor vision development or large differences in the prescription of the two eyes could be the source of the complaint.

Headaches

Headaches can be caused by a myriad of physical problems. Eyestrain is just one of these possibilities, but it should be the first thing ruled out when a child complains of headaches. In particular, eyestrain-related headaches tend to happen more toward the end of the day, develop in the temples or forehead area, and possibly occur less frequently on weekends or during vacations.

Nausea or Dizziness

These symptoms are rare, but if they do occur, they could easily result from an internalization of a visual misalignment of the eyes. The visual system and the vestibular (balance) systems are connected. You can experience this connection when standing on one foot with eyes open and staring a one point. Once you close your eyes, you will likely fall over within a few seconds.

Tiring Quickly while Reading

Muscles around the eyes control convergence, or turning in, of the eyes toward a near object. When these muscles become easily fatigued, the condition is known as *convergence insufficiency*, and tiring is the most obvious complaint. The good news is that this condition is treated easily with a program of vision therapy. (See Chapter 11 on page 141 for some of these techniques).

Learning Disabilities

The signs that follow can all be attributable to vision problems, but they may also indicate that your child has a learning disability—from being hyperactive to having dyslexia. If your child's eyesight is found to be normal but these signs persist, consider talking to your pediatrician or a learning specialist.

Short Attention Span for Reading

This symptom often occurs with tiring of the eyes. The typical cause of this is poor eye coordination, which is trainable in most children. This may also indicate a learning disability, which makes reading very difficult.

The Irlen Method and Dyslexia

Researchers continue to investigate the role of the visual system in *dyslexia,* which may be defined as an inability to read and understand written language despite having normal intelligence. The visual system is almost certainly involved in some way with the problem, although exactly how it is involved is not clear. Dyslexic children usually have good visual acuity, although they seem to have difficulty focusing their eyes. Interestingly, children with severe strabismus (crossed eyes or walleyes) usually do not have difficulty reading because they manage to suppress the image from the severely affected eye and read with the good eye. Children with mild strabismus, on the other hand, may seem to be dyslexic because they struggle to fuse the two different images from their two eyes. This is not true dyslexia, but rather a binocular vision problem that may mimic dyslexic symptoms.

In the 1980s, education specialist Helen Irlen found another cause associated with dyslexia. Her findings suggest that at least some dyslexics are extremely sensitive to light. She named this disorder scotopic sensitivity syndrome (SSS). To assist persons with SSS, Irlen developed a treatment using special light-filtering colored lenses, now called Irlen lenses. While not widely accepted in the eyecare community, Irlen's theory is an interesting concept that is receiving more study in the area of learning disability.

Although there is no cure for dyslexia, dyslexic individuals can learn to read and write with appropriate education or treatment. Some research evidence indicates that specialized phonics instruction can help remediate the reading deficits. The fundamental aim is to make children aware of the relationships between what they see on the page and the sound of the language, and to associate these relationships with reading and spelling. It has been found that training that is focused on both visual language and oral expression yields longer-lasting gains than mere oral training. The key in this context is to realize that symptoms of dyslexia are often similar to symptoms of a visual disorder, so ruling out the visual component is critical to avoid a lifelong label that may not be appropriate for particular children.

Poor Reading Comprehension

Reading is only effective if the reader can understand the material that is being read. Ask your child to read a few paragraphs and then ask your child to stop and tell you what he or she feels the material means. Children who put too much effort into controlling their eyes will not be able to comprehend the material they are reading.

Loss of Place

Since the eye muscles are moving the eyes so quickly, the eyes may lose their place and then the words will be mixed up and not make any sense. This issue occurs most often at the end of a line in text.

Frequent Omission of Words

It is unlikely that we read the words on a page one word at a time. Our eyes typically pick up the shape of the word and then the brain recalls likely similar words and makes sense of the sentence. If the eye muscles are not moving the eyes correctly, they will skip over some words and the sentence will not make sense.

Writing Uphill or Downhill

Our horizontal eye movements develop earlier than our vertical eye movements. When there is a deficiency in one of these systems, this hand-eye coordination dysfunction will occur.

Rereading or Skipping Lines Unknowingly

As with any eye-tracking process, smooth eye movements are required. If a child has not learned to coordinate the eyes effortlessly, inaccurate movements will lead to skipping lines or rereading the same line.

Failure to Visualize What Is Read

This problem speaks to visual perception, which first requires that the eyes be already trained to move smoothly across the page.

Repeated Confusion over Left-Right Directions

As strange as it may seem, proper visual development depends upon an infant's repeated crawling pattern. This crawling leads to a correct detection of right vs. left in viewing objects. Sometime children need to relearn how to tell right-left directions in order to learn visual perception.

This A-B-C-D list covers most of the general observations you will see for eyestrain-related reading issues. Some of the behavioral issues may vary, as all kids are slightly different. Getting a complete eye examination, which includes testing of vision at reading distance, will rule out vision as a source of difficulty in any child who has difficulty with schoolwork. As you will see, how your child performs in school may be an important key in judging whether or not your child has a vision problem.

VISION PROBLEMS BY GRADE

Vision problems can develop at any age, but there do seem to be certain times during a child's schooling when they are more likely to occur. Second grade, fourth grade, seventh grade, and ninth grade are key years in which to pay special attention to your child's vision development.

Second Grade

In second grade, there is often a sudden increase in nearsightedness among students. This increase may be the result of second grade being the time when children generally learn to read. In addition, the demand for close work greatly increases over previous school years in second grade.

Fourth Grade

In fourth grade, instead of learning to read, children begin reading to learn. This presents the possibility that a not fully mastered skill must be used to investigate new areas of knowledge. It is as if you had just begun to learn French and suddenly had to study nuclear physics in this language. The result of this kind of stress, and of the even more intense close work, is often nearsightedness. Sometimes a child will just quit trying and become an underachiever.

Seventh Grade

In seventh grade, children are in the heart of middle school. The physical growth spurt they experience combined with the tremendously increased demand for near-point work is a recipe for nearsightedness.

Ninth Grade

In ninth grade, the reading assignments pile up and the pressures to achieve increase. Teenagers may adapt to this stress by developing near-sightedness (if they have not done so already). If vision problems go uncorrected, teenagers may give up on schoolwork and show declining achievement, or even turn to juvenile delinquency.

KEEP YOUR EYES OPEN

All these periods of high stress require a good vision examination, which is suggested every year. Therefore, when September rolls around and you buy new clothes and school supplies for your child and make appointments for medical examinations and dental checkups, do not forget about the one school need that must be in the best working order: your child's vision. In addition, please remember that school vision screenings are not a substitute for a complete visual examination.

Eyestrain can occur at any age, gender, or level of education. We hope and assume that a normally developing child has a visual system that grows and develops properly. Nature does not always follow the rules, though, and deficiencies can arise. By catching your child's vision problem early, you can help your child to avoid the stress of struggling to read and write.

Just keep in mind that there are three options available to working with a visual system that needs assistance. The first is to work on a program of vision therapy that trains the visual system to perform optimally. Secondly, eyeglasses may be worn—either for occasional reading or for other specific visual tasks. Thirdly, both methods may be employed simultaneously. Wearing eyeglasses is not the end of the world for children (of any age) or adults. Many times, they assist the visual system in getting better, either with or without therapy. While many might call them "crutches," remember that crutches most often temporarily assist the body so it can heal. In the next chapter, we will discuss different lens colors and configurations, and how each accomplishes the task of reducing eyestrain.

5

Maybe It's Your Glasses?

The general belief is that eyestrain is the result of poor vision, but research indicates there are many more factors at work. For example, maybe you have good vision but are now using your eyes in awkward conditions—poor lighting, terrible ergonomics with your computer, or other situations that strain your vision. Simply put, for the majority of us, the accuracy of our eyesight decreases over time. If you have had 20/20 vision since you were a child, you may have noticed that you now squint a little when you are reading or when you look at something at a distance. That additional effort to focus may be the cause of your eyestrain—and it is probably time to visit an eye specialist to get a pair of glasses. In addition, of course, if you already wear glasses but seem to be squinting to see well, the same advice goes for you.

Interestingly enough, the first wearable glasses go back to the thirteenth century. The Italians created glass-blown lenses and inserted them into wooden frames. Of course, it was rather hit or miss as to how well these glasses improved a person's sight, but they must have worked well enough to be used throughout the next seven centuries. Today, the science of creating lenses that restore more accurate sight has come a long way. There are now over six million different combinations of powers and hundreds of different designs of lenses to help reduce eyestrain. In this chapter we will look at some of the lenses that might work best for your situation and, in doing so, may likely put an end to your eyestrain.

SINGLE VISION

The single-vision lens is the simplest design because there is only one power throughout the entire surface of the lens. It can accommodate for farsighted, nearsighted, and astigmatism prescriptions. With this lens, vision should be clear almost all the way to the very edge of the lens, not simply through the optical center, which is the spot that you would look through most (for distance vision). The prescription in the lens is typically for long-distance viewing, with the crystalline lens within the eye actively focusing for near viewing tasks.

For nearsighted prescriptions, the lens is thicker on the edges and thinner in the center, thus "weakening" light rays that pass through to the eye. The issue with nearsighted eyes is that they are too "long," so light normally focuses too soon. Weakening the focusing power of light will allow it to focus further back onto the retina.

In reality, this type of prescription tends to get stronger every year or so. The issue arises that, while the light is now focusing on the retina, the person is still using their eyes improperly and straining. This could happen several ways, from simple overuse at a close reading distance to reading in poor lighting or watching TV or computers too closely. These situations create an over-focusing of the lens, which results in eyestrain. Thus, the eyes will continue to strain and adapt by making it easier to see up close (thus, nearsightedness) at the expense of clear distant vision.

For farsighted prescriptions, the corrective lens is thicker at the center and thinner at the edges. This design serves to increase the bending of light to focus sooner, given that farsighted eyes are "shorter." This farsighted prescription, since it achieves the same purpose as the crystalline lens within, can take over some of the work so that internal lens does not need to work as hard. For this reason, these stress-relieving lenses allow the eyes to relax more, which in turn will relieve eyestrain.

One caveat in using this type of lens is that it might seem that you become more dependent on them. Once you start using this lens to reduce eyestrain, your eyes will feel better. When you remove them, your eyes may feel strained again! This happens because the muscles inside your eye relax when viewing through the lens. When called upon to act again without the lenses, they will need to work harder again. Think of your exercise program. If you exercise regularly, the workout does not cause any pain or discomfort. If you take a break for an extended period and then begin to work out again, you feel the pain in the muscles that next day. If a doctor prescribes lenses properly, they should allow you to work without eyestrain. Performing some of the eye techniques at the end of this book (see Chapter 11 on page 141) should help you to maintain well-performing eye muscles.

For astigmatism prescriptions, the lenses are curved so that the prescription in the vertical direction and the prescription in the horizontal direction are different. This would correspond to the powers in your eye in each of those directions. You will recall that astigmatism is an optical distortion where the horizontal and vertical prescriptions are different, typically corresponding to the curvatures of the cornea. Some describe this as "football-shaped," which illustrates the different curves in different directions, flat in one direction and steeper in the other.

Due to the different curvatures, the light entering the eye will be distorted, with no single point of focus. (The word originates from the Latin *a-stigma*, which means "without point.") Thus, an eye with astigmatism will attempt to focus continually back-and-forth, trying to find a clear point of focus. This is one of the most common causes of eyestrain. Once an optician grinds the proper prescription into a single-vision lens, the light can focus properly at one point on the retina and vision will be clear. The lenses must be fit accurately in the frame because the person must look directly through that optical center when viewing distance vision in order to maintain clarity. Again, the viewing of near objects would be accomplished by the crystalline lens within the eye, but at least there would be a clear point of light on which to focus.

BIFOCAL LENSES

Back in 1824, Benjamin Franklin realized that he needed two different powers in his glasses—one to see clearly at a distance and another to see clearly at a near distance (a case of presbyopia). He also realized that when he was reading his books his eyes were in a lower viewing position. He cleverly cut the two lenses in half and glued the reading portion at the bottom of the distance portion, thus creating the first *bifocal lens*. It was not until the beginning of the twentieth century that technology allowed for heated fusing of the two halves and created a fully functional bifocal lens. These lenses had a visible line that demarcated the power difference between the two lenses, which had some optical challenges ("image jump" due to power differences being a major one).

Several further developments in bifocal lenses quickly followed, some with rounded segments for reading, and others with a "flat-top" design (like a sideways "D"). Since the segment for reading was typically smaller (making reading more challenging) a more recent development was the executive bifocal, which had a line all the way across the lens, allowing for a much wider reading zone. The transition, however, from distance to near reading created a more significant difference in the image, so the eyes had to adjust. This was a challenge for the older reader and caused severe eyestrain issues.

One other significant configuration of the bifocal concerns the height of the lower portion. If the top of the bifocal is placed too high in the lens, it will interfere with distance and intermediate-distance viewing. If placed too low, then the person will have to raise his or her chin too high to read at a traditional reading distance. Fitting the lens is an art as much as it is a science.

TRIFOCALS

Bifocals are adequate for the majority of people with a need for both distance and near corrections. Most people's eyes can focus for intermediate activities—such as computer work, card playing, music reading, seeing prices on grocery shelves, or working at a large desk—by using either the distance-lens or near-lens segment of their glasses. But some people need special lenses for this intermediate, arm's-length distance. The answer for these people is—you guessed it—trifocals. A *trifocal lens* corrects vision at three different focal distances.

The first trifocals were developed in the 1940s and were similar in design to the flat-top bifocals. The only difference was that trifocals had a third lens segment, for intermediate vision, inserted between the near and distance segments. The fitting of these lenses was extremely difficult. The intermediate segment needed to be low enough so the wearer could look comfortably through the distance segment while driving, but it also needed to be high enough so the wearer could look comfortably through the reading segment at, for example, groceries on a supermarket shelf while keeping the head in a normal position. Not surprisingly, few people adapted to the first trifocals.

PROGRESSIVE ADDITION LENSES (PALS)

Although first patented in 1907, it was not until the early 1950s that the first modern design of a *progressive addition lens* (PAL) reached the market. PALs are characterized by a gradient change of power throughout the viewing portion of the lens, allowing clear distant vision through the top, intermediate vision through the middle, and near vision in the lower section. There are blurred sections of the lens off to the periphery.

All powers are available for PALs: nearsighted, farsighted, and astigmatism. The fitting of this lens is critical (and cannot be done properly online) and depends on many factors, including the overall purpose of the lens (generally distance or near viewing), posture, and height of the person, as well as some other lifestyle factors. If someone is looking through the wrong portion of a PAL, this person will adjust his or her head, neck, shoulders or back to accommodate for imperfect vision, therefore causing more physical strain than eyestrain. Remember that the eyes lead the body, so if the eyes cannot see properly, the affected person will naturally adjust body posture to reduce strain on the eyes.

While mistakenly called "no-line bifocals" (actually PALs), there are over 80 million people wearing them, and there are now close to 300 different designs of the lens. Some have wider reading zones, while

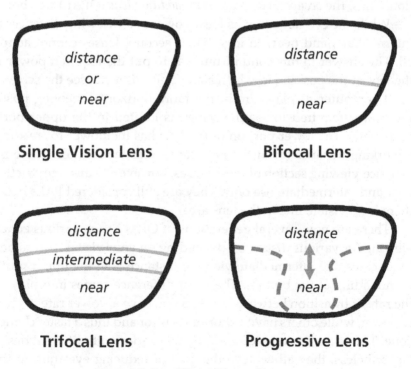

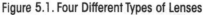

Figure 5.1. Four Different Types of Lenses

others have wider intermediate zones or other technical modifications. Now there are digitally manufactured lenses that put some of the power on the front of the lens and some on the back, designed to slim down the profile of the lens, making it thinner and lighter.

OCCUPATIONAL PROGRESSIVE ADDITION LENSES (OPALS)

In Chapter 3, we learned about the challenges of viewing computer displays over reading material on paper. We can be confident that Ben Franklin did not have computer displays in mind when he designed the first bifocal lenses.

Due to the unique viewing situation of computer displays, PAL users complained of neck and back aches after using a computer for short periods. Recall that the lower viewing range is for reading on a desktop and computer displays are higher in the visual field. The solution is to make special lenses that can accommodate this unique viewing situation. Thus, the *occupational progressive addition lens* (OPAL) was born.

While the eye can adapt its focal power to all viewing distances (far, intermediate, and near) in less than a second, lenses cannot adapt at all. The answer to this conundrum was to put the required power into the lens at the position in which a computer user can see the screen. As most computer displays are in the more horizontal viewing posture, the power required to see the screen is located in the upper portion of the lens. The lower portion of the lens has the power for reading at a working distance (or at the keyboard) of sixteen inches. There is no distance-viewing section of these lenses, however, so they are strictly for near and intermediate use only. They are still considered PALs because there is no visible line in the lens area.

There are now several generations of OPALs with various zones of viewing for various distances, depending on your visual requirements. In all cases, the intermediate-viewing distance is in the upper portion, with reading at the bottom. The main difference comes into play with the rate of transition between zones. Some have a slower rate of change of power, while others have a shorter corridor and thus a faster changing zone. The width of zones of viewing also varies with different designs. Nevertheless, they all achieve the goal of reducing eyestrain in those people who look at computer displays.

LENS MATERIALS

For nearly seven hundred years, lenses used to correct vision were made of glass, which is why we call them eyeglasses. So, while the frames they came in may have changed with the advancement of technology and, of course, fashion, the lenses themselves remained the same—that is up until the late 1950s. Since then, optical lenses have changed greatly due to the development of specialized plastics.

CR-39 Lens

This material originated during World War II, and since then it has been further refined to improve its optical properties. *CR-39* plastic soon became the standard lens material in about 80 percent of American lens prescriptions. Its main advantage over glass is its weight, being about half the weight of a glass lens per diopter (a unit of measurement of the optical power of a lens). This fact makes these lenses more comfortable to wear, especially for people with high prescriptions, regardless of power.

Plastic also offers much more protection for the eyes. The lens can still be broken, but it takes a much greater force to break it. For rimless frames, plastic lenses are a much better choice than glass because they do not chip at the exposed edges nearly as easily. In addition, plastic does not splinter into tiny slivers like glass. Finally plastic lenses may be tinted different colors using a hot-dying procedure. (Glass requires a color coating on the surface).

Polycarbonate Lens

In 1985, a new kind of plastic lens called a *polycarbonate* lens entered the market, and it has proven to have some advantages over the CR-39 lens. The density of this plastic allows it to be formed into lenses that are much thinner than lenses made of CR-39 plastic, and yet these lenses can achieve equal optical power. Polycarbonate lenses are also half the weight of conventional plastic lenses, offer inherent ultraviolet protection, and may be treated to be scratch-resistant. One of the most impressive properties of polycarbonate plastic is that it is practically unbreakable. A twelve-gauge shotgun fired at a polycarbonate lens at close range will only dent it! It is obviously the ideal material to use for protective eyewear. The only drawback is that the usable optical zone (the part through which you see) of polycarbonate lenses is slightly narrower than that of conventional plastic lenses, so distortions can occur in peripheral vision when made in the higher prescriptions. This issue can cause significant eyestrain. Here's a fun fact: This polycarbonate material is also used to make jet fighter cockpits.

High-Index Plastic

Adding to the choices now is a high-density plastic known as "high-index plastic." The term "index" refers to the density of the lens, which can affect the way it bends light. This plastic is similar to CR-39 plastic, except it is denser (even more dense than polycarbonate), allowing lenses to be made thinner and lighter. The chief disadvantage of CR-39, polycarbonate, and high-index plastics is that they can become scratched more easily than glass. A scratch-resistant coating, however, can be applied to plastic lenses to reduce their susceptibility to scratches. A scratch-resistant coating is necessary on a plastic lens, and is usually included in the cost. Although scratch-resistant coating is very effective, it does not approximate the hardness of glass.

Glass

Glass lenses are still available and do have certain advantages. If you have a mild prescription and a frame that is not very large, the weight of the lenses may not be a problem. For someone whose glasses are just for occasional reading, glass lenses might do the trick. They are more scratch-resistant than plastic, and they have an inherent ability to block out UV light. There is also a new version of glass that simulates some of the properties of high-index plastic, forming thinner, lighter glass lenses that are scratch-resistant.

LENS TREATMENTS

Eyeglass lenses can have certain treatments added to them, or included in them as part of the material of the lenses themselves. These treatments add to the features that make lenses either more durable or protective for the wearer, and might even help to relieve eyestrain under certain conditions.

Anti-Scratch Coating

As described earlier, lenses made from plastic rather than glass are soft enough to require a coating on them to reduce the likelihood of scratching. If everyone took care of their glasses, which means cleaned and stored properly in their cases every time they removed them, it is unlikely that this coating would be necessary. In real life, however, this is rarely the case. Thus, an anti-scratch coating is routinely applied to lenses to harden their exterior surfaces. In most situations, this coating should be included in the price of lenses.

Anti-Reflective Coating

In photographs, have you ever noticed that you can see the lenses of the people wearing glasses but not their eyes? This effect is due to the light in the room or sunlight being reflected off the front surface of the glasses. This occurs because only 92 percent of light passes through a lens. Of the remaining 8 percent, 4 percent bounces off the front surface and another 4 percent bounces off the back. An anti-reflective lens coating can take care of this problem, allowing over 99 percent of light through the lens.

The coating has some distinct advantages. With an anti-reflective coating on the lenses, other people can see the wearer's eyes through the

Night Vision

Many of us have given up on driving when the sun goes down. It seems our eyes cannot see the road in front of us very well when it gets dark. As it turns out, poor night vision may certainly be associated with aging, but it can affect people at any age. It can be due to a number of reasons, such as the fact that our pupils get larger at night, which can blur the view at a normal driving distance. In addition, our rods, which are responsible for night vision, are not located in the central part of the retina, where the sharpest vision is centered. By using an anti-reflective coating on lenses, more light will pass through the lenses, thus keeping light from scattering and obscuring your night vision.

lenses and sometimes not perceive at all that lenses are in the frames. Some people consider this a major cosmetic advantage, especially if they wear one of the higher prescriptions, which occasionally cause rings of reflected light to be visible in the lenses. People who drive at night appreciate the coating because it eliminates the glare from oncoming headlights. The one disadvantage of having anti-reflective coating on the lenses of your glasses is that they tend to smudge and need special cleaning and handling, although newer technology seems to be addressing this issue.

Ultraviolet Coating

Lenses can also be treated with a coating that blocks ultraviolet, or UV, light. Ultraviolet light is the highest energy level of light that reaches the eye, but the cornea and crystalline lens absorb most of it. Some authorities believe cataracts to be the result of the absorption of UV light by the crystalline lens inside the eye over many years. Plastic lenses require treatment with a special coating to block out UV light, whereas glass lenses inherently block most UV light without the need of any coating.

A UV coating is especially handy for sunglasses, but if you spend a lot of time indoors, there is limited exposure to UV light (the small amount from fluorescent lights is negligible). When computers first hit the market, there was concern about the UV light being emitted from the display, but this concern was unfounded, as the amount of UV light encountered from the screen diminished significantly at a distance of four inches, and most of the UV light was actually found at the back of the display rather than in front of it.

Coating to Block Blue Light

While the cornea and crystalline lens absorb ultraviolet light, the adjacent blue light passes through these structures and reaches the retina. Until recently, it was not an issue for eye health or eyestrain. When computer displays were made with light-emitting diode (LED) lights, however, studies were conducted to see if this type of light caused problems.

When looking at the spectrum of light produced by LEDs, scientists noted that the light had high intensity in the blue light region of the spectrum. A coating that blocks blue light can be incorporated into lenses, but most likely it will give the lenses a slightly yellow tint. We will review the science and some of the concerns of blue light in the next chapter.

Photochromic Lenses

Glass lenses were the first lenses available as photochromic lenses, which react to light and automatically tint to become dark lenses as the surrounding light gets brighter, such as when you move from indoors to a sunny outdoor environment. The photochromic process is not a coating, since the darkening material is in the matrix of the lens. Today, plastic lenses that react to light are also available. Plastic photochromic lenses darken in bright light but do not get as dark as glass photochromic lenses.

When it comes to tinted glasses in general, ordinary tinting does not work as well in glass lenses as it does in plastic lenses. It is not as uniform in glass in higher prescriptions as it is in plastic. When choosing tinted plastic lenses, it is important to know that polycarbonate lenses do not tint as dark as other plastics.

Sports with Glasses

Today's glass lenses are tempered (required by federal law) to minimize splintering, but they are still not as safe as polycarbonate plastic lenses, so I do not recommend wearing any glasses with glass lenses when playing sports.

SUNGLASSES

Standard sunglasses that do not change color are available off the rack in almost any drug or department store. The optical properties of the lenses in these glasses, however, are typically subpar, and may lead to eyestrain. If the lenses are not optical quality—i.e., ground and polished like prescription glasses—then there can be distortions in the lenses, or the intensity of the color of the lenses may not be dark enough to prevent glare. Good-quality lenses and properly fitting frames can make your eyes feel relaxed. You can purchase good-quality sunglasses from a professional optical shop or optometrist's office.

A mirror coating applied to sunglass lenses will further decrease the transmission of light through the lenses. Sunglass lenses can also be polarized, which is a technique that blocks the scattering of light. One way to visualize polarization is to think of someone holding one end of a jump rope and spinning it in a circular motion. This is essentially how light travels: in all directions from a point source. Now, imagine there is a picket fence between the attachment of the rope and the person twirling it. As the person twirls the rope in a circular motion, the rope simply goes up and down due to the restrictions of the fence. This is what polarization does: It restricts the light to one direction, which serves to reduce scattering and reflections. This is most visible in nature when looking at water from a boat or shoreline. Light from the sun and sky will reflect off the water and make it difficult to see through the water. With polarized sunglasses, however, you can view into the water and see below the surface. Thus, if you plan to spend a significant time around water, polarized sunglasses are the best option to see without inducing any eyestrain.

CHOOSING LENSES

So, which is the best lens for you? Discuss the different lens materials and coatings with your optometrist or optician. Find out what is included in the price of your glasses, and what best suits your needs. If you just need to wear glasses occasionally for reading, then glass may be the best way to go. If you wear glasses on a full-time basis but your prescription is not very high, then CR-39 plastic will do nicely. If your prescription is not very high or you are in a high-risk environment for breakage, polycarbonate or high-index plastic is for you. For kids, who are always tough on glasses, polycarbonate is your best option, since it is the safest way to go. Glass will certainly last longer and not become as badly scratched, but polycarbonate is much safer. For a quick comparison of glass, CR-39, polycarbonate, and high-index lenses, see Table 5.1 on page 63.

Table 5.1. Comparison of Different Lens Materials				
Lens Type	Glass	CR-39 Plastic	Polycarbonate Plastic	High-Index Plastic
Weight	Heavy	Light	Very light	Very light
Impact Resistance	Fair	Good	Excellent	Good
Tintability	Fair	Excellent	Good	Excellent
UV Protection	Excellent (inherent ability)	Poor (can be treated)	Excellent (inherent ability)	Poor (can be treated)
Scratch Resistance	Excellent	Fair	Fair	Fair
Thickness per Given Power	Thick	Thicker	Very thin	Thinnest
Available as Photochromic Lens?	Yes	Yes	Yes	Yes
Suitable for Rimless Frames?	No	Yes, in lower prescriptions. No, in higher prescriptions.	Yes	Yes

CONTACT LENSES

With the remarkable development and growth of contact lens technology, contact lenses have exploded in popularity. There are now over 40 million Americans wearing contact lenses on a regular basis. Contacts are available for almost any type of vision correction, including near-sightedness, farsightedness, astigmatism, and multifocal astigmatism conditions. They also offer eye color-changing options and even photochromic lenses.

When soft contact lenses initially became available on a commercial basis in the early 1970s, there were significant challenges in making these lenses comfortable for a full-day wearing schedule, as well as difficulties in having them last for a full year. The previously available "hard" contact lenses would typically last for several years, but soft lenses tore or attracted deposits onto the lens surface, creating an uncomfortable foreign-body sensation. This issue led to blurred and distorted images, which, of course, led to eyestrain.

As technology and acceptance of soft lenses continued to develop, these contacts became less expensive and more disposable. Instead of lasting for a full year, replacement of the lenses was on a quarterly basis, and then eventually became monthly. Today we have soft lenses that wearers remove and throw away after just one day of wear. This type of lens is the most comfortable and healthiest choice when it comes to wearing contact lenses.

When computers started to make their way into the corporate workplace, many contact lens wearers had to resort to wearing glasses again during their workdays, typically due to their lenses drying out toward the end of the day. The cause of this problem was a combination of lens deposits and a decrease in blinking by the computer user. Now most people can comfortably wear their contact lenses throughout their workdays without irritation or discomfort. If you experience dryness or eyestrain using contact lenses, a visit to an eyecare professional is warranted. Many times a change of cleaning solution, a new contact-lens care regimen, or switching to a different brand of lenses will resolve the issue.

CONCLUSION

Now you know there are many options for compensating for poor or strained vision. Given all the possibilities, it is important to discuss your work habits, your work environment, your computer use, your hobbies, and any other situation in which you use your eyes with your eyecare professional. In addition, it is also important to realize that our various viewing conditions may not be able to be resolved with just one pair of glasses. Could you golf any entire golf course using just one club? Moreover, how many pair of shoes does the average person own? One pair will obviously not be appropriate for all occasions. Thus, be open to using different pairs of glasses to compensate for numerous viewing conditions, thus ensuring you will be able to see clearly and comfortably at all times.

In the next chapter, we will look at various viewing situations that can be stressful for your eyes and lead to eyestrain.

6

Lighting

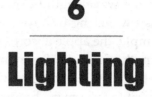

It has been said, "Without light, there is no sight." This adage proves true because the ability to see is dependent on the amount and quality of light that enters our eyes. The retina consists of rods and cones, which are specialized cells that detect light and dark, as well as about seven million colors. Given our modern day visual tasks, it is not surprising that we are pushing our visual abilities to their limits.

In the previous chapter, we discussed the different options for adjusting the focusing of light, and how to enhance our vision with lenses. Now we can review how we see in various lighting conditions, whether they are located in the workplace or at home. There are continual modifications and enhancements in the lighting world, and these affect the conditions in which we work. Moreover, they all have their advantages and challenges. Let us look at how lighting affects our eyesight.

LIGHTING BASICS

Before we can talk about vision, we will need to go over some basics about the nature of light. When light rays come from a source of light, they radiate from the light in a similar fashion to the waves formed in water when a rock hits its surface. Light waves travel in various lengths, and the unit of length used to measure waves of light is the *nanometer* (nan-AHM-iter), which refers to one millionth of a millimeter, or one billionth of a meter.

The range of light visible to the human eye is called the "visible spectrum," which describes light with a wavelength of between 400 and 700 nanometers (nm) approximately. Ultraviolet light is not visible to humans because it has a wavelength below 400 nm, and neither is infrared light, which has a wavelength above 700 nm. When white light hits a red apple, for example, the apple absorbs all the light rays except for those with a wavelength of about 650 nanometers, which it reflects. Humans have learned to call this particular wavelength of reflected light "red." Each color visible to humans has its own wavelength. Blue is about 460 nanometers, green about 520 nanometers, and yellow about 575 nanometers, and so on. When we perceive a colored object, what we see is that part of the light spectrum that is being reflected and reaching our eyes.

COLOR BLINDNESS

For approximately 8 percent of men and 0.5 percent of women in the United States (these statistics vary somewhat by country), something goes wrong with color perception. The color-connection mechanism does not work properly, and these people are often referred to as color blind. Actually, the term "color blind" is a misnomer, as nearly every person with this affliction has only a deficiency, not a total absence, in his or her ability to see a full range of colors. It is possible to have excellent (i.e., 20/20) vision and still have a color deficiency, which is the term I prefer.

The retina contains several million cones that are responsible for perception of color. There are three basic types of cones in the retina: one that processes blue, one that processes red, and one that processes green. People who are color deficient may be missing a certain type of color cone in their retinas, or their cones may be deficient in their ability to process color signals. When the red-receiving cones do not function properly or are absent, the person will have a defect in the perception of the color red. The technical term for "red blindness" is *protanopia* (proh-tan-OH-pee-ah). When the green-receiving cones are not functioning or are absent, there will be "green blindness," which is called *deuteranopia* (doo-ter-an-OH-pee-ah). Deficiencies in perceiving yellows and blues also occur, but they are extremely rare.

Although color deficiency can be acquired during a person's life due to certain diseases or as a side effect of certain drugs, it is more often genetically inherited and present from birth. Men are about fifteen times more likely to be color deficient than are women because of the way in which color deficiency is inherited.

An eye doctor can quickly and simply test color vision. If it is determined that you have some form of color deficiency, fear not. Color problems do not affect visual acuity, and even the most color-deficient person can have 20/20 vision. If you want to be an electrical worker or a pilot, you probably need excellent color discrimination, but a color deficiency can be coped with in most occupations. Of course, it can be inconvenient. One of my patients said that she always knew when her color-deficient coworker had had a disagreement with his wife—he would come to work in clothes that clashed.

Color deficiency does not involve any real eye disease or aberration in the clarity of eyesight, so the treatment of color deficiency is very limited. Most often, it consists of making a note in the affected patients eye doctor's chart, making sure the patient is aware of the problem and counseling the patient to be cautious of taking jobs that require accurate color matching.

Color Blindness Breakthrough?

EnChroma is the product name of a lens that has shown to effectively manage color deficiency in some cases, enhancing color perception. Originally, doctors performing laser surgery used these lenses during the procedures. The coating on these lenses enhanced the wavelengths of light, allowing doctors to view the laser beams more accurately. What they discovered was that it also made colors look more vivid. When used by color-deficient individuals, the lenses did something unexpected: They enhanced color—not for everyone, but for some.

Most types of color blindness occur when there is an excessive overlap of green and red color cones in the eye, causing distinct hues to become indistinguishable. As a result, the number of shades of color a typical color-deficient person can see may be reduced by as much as 90 percent. EnChroma lens technology selectively filters out wavelengths of light at the precise point at which confusion or excessive overlap of color sensitivity occurs. The green and red cones are altered in such a way that there is a greater amount of difference in color discrimination along the so-called "confusion line" for the affected individual. Contact information for EnChroma is listed in the Resources on page 167.

READING AND COLOR VISION

While most people feel that 20/20 vision is the standard in healthy eyes, it is far from the only issue to address. Any child who displays a learning issue in school needs an examination from a developmental optometrist to determine how visual perception occurs. The most complex eye problems are in children with 20/20 vision!

To optimize reading, there must be high contrast between the color of the letters and the background of the paper. Black letters on a white background offer the highest contrast, making this the preferred printing for reading material, but not everyone is able to view this configuration with optimal performance. Many children who have reading challenges may actually have a visual dysfunction caused by the high contrast between the letters and background of their reading materials. This condition has been studied and found to be more common than formerly believed.

Irlen Lenses

In the 1980s, Dr. Helen Irlen, a psychologist, developed a theory that at least some dyslexic people have an unusual sensitivity to light that interferes with their reading ability. According to Dr. Irlen's theory, these people use their night vision all the time, which creates some visual distortion when they try to read black letters on a white background. Irlen named this problem *scotopic sensitivity syndrome* (SSS).

In an effort to find a way to help people with SSS, Dr. Irlen experimented with colored light-filtering lenses to use while reading. These lenses are now called "Irlen lenses." The approach used by the Irlen Institute is to give the patient a complete vision examination first to rule out any refractive problems—that is, make sure the patient can see clearly. Next, an evaluation is made to determine the exact visual distortions experienced relating to light sensitivity, visual resolution (blurring), span of focus, and sustained focus during the reading process. Lastly, lenses are designed to minimize or eliminate the distortions, using the appropriate tint from among 150 different color possibilities. Dr. Irlen's process has created some controversy in the medical community. A few studies have looked at the concept and methods of Irlen lenses and most have concluded that there is no consistent evidence that Irlen therapy improves reading comprehension in dyslexic people. A placebo effect may be present in some studies that support Irlen therapy. More likely there are underlying vision problems that are responsible for the symptoms experienced by candidates for Irlen filters. For more information on the Irlen method and Irlen lenses, see Dr. Irlen's published works or write to the Irlen Institite. (See Resources on page 167.)

Clinical research has confirmed that blue filters have a significant positive impact on reading comprehension in reading disabled children but not in normal readers, (the study was conducted with children in grades four through six). One study showed that 87 percent of the reading disabled children showed an improvement in comprehension that averaged 45 percent when using the blue filter. While this result is limited to blue filters, it suggests a visual-processing component to this condition and lends credence to the work done by Dr. Irlen.

PRINT VS. ELECTRONIC DISPLAYS

As far back as the fifteenth century, we have been using paper as a print medium. Paper technology has obviously changed considerably, but the basic concept of applying ink to paper has been with us for quite a while. With the advent of computer displays, however, our viewing of text has changed radically, and likely not for the better. Let us review the differences in the printing on paper as opposed to electronic displays.

Reading text on paper requires light to reflect from the page and into the eyes. Thus, location of lighting in the room where reading takes place is critical to clarity and comfort for the reader. There are several types of lighting, as defined by the Illuminating Engineering Society of North America (IESNA), the group that sets the standards for lighting. The purpose of this not-for-profit organization is to communicate information on all aspects of good lighting practices, both in business and professional settings. Most lighting and interior designers are well aware of these standards and incorporate them into the design of living and working spaces.

How you set up an office or workspace for reading has many variables. The one aspect of lighting to maximize reading is to assure that light is reflected from the page into your eyes properly. The ideal location of this light would be slightly behind your head and a bit off to the side, so that you do not cast a shadow on the reading material. To see if you have your lighting properly positioned, simply take a pocket mirror and lay it on top of your reading material. If you see the reflection of the light bulb in the mirror, it is causing too much glare and the light should be shifted.

In most of these viewing situations, the book or paper is in a lowered viewing angle, where you are slightly lowering your head but mostly lowering your eyes to view the material. This is a normal reading posture. Excessive lowering of the head will cause strain on the neck or shoulders and lead to discomfort. Your line of sight should be perpendicular to the angle of the book.

Computer displays offer a completely different configuration. First, the letters are generated by pixels, which are very minute sources of light behind the display screen. It is beyond the scope of this book to delve into the technology behind this configuration, but let us just say that the dots on the screen are not typically as refined as printed letters on paper.

With this being said, newer technology in display screens is making the difference less obvious with each generation of display. Most desktop displays, however, are still configured to be more vertically oriented, so you are looking more straight ahead when viewing the text. This is not a natural posture for the eyes to maintain for an extended period. When looking at a near object, the line of sight of each eye must turn in toward each other—a process called convergence. The convergence of the two eyes toward each other must coordinate with the focusing of the crystalline lens within the eyes, which are controlled by a different set of muscles. Studies show that focusing is most accurate in viewing a close object in a lower posture rather than in a straight-ahead or upward posture. Thus, we should slightly lower the computer display so we can maintain a lower viewing posture.

Where lighting is concerned, it is important that we have uniform lighting to avoid high contrast in our field of view. The IESNA recommendation suggests that the background of the computer display and the surrounding 25 degrees to either side be approximately equal in illumination. This is one rationale for not watching TV in the dark.

Another aspect of electronic displays is the fact that they are now available in "full color." In fact, most displays tout an ability to offer over 16 million colors! This fact sounds quite impressive until you consider that the human eye can only perceive about half that many. Nevertheless, it is imperative that you adjust the colors of your display to maximize the contrast on the screen (to make the letters stand out) while moderating the screen's brightness so it matches room lighting.

BLUE LIGHT BLUES

At the beginning of this chapter, we briefly discussed the electromagnetic spectrum that contains all the colors of the rainbow that make up white light. The sun contains a full spectrum of all these colors, but different types of lighting contain differing amounts colors, with some occurring in to a greater degree than others. For example, if you look at a standard light bulb, you will notice that it appears somewhat yellowish in color, whereas a fluorescent bulb has much more of a blue tint to it. Different types of lighting typically allow different colors of the spectrum to predominate.

The retina of the eye is most sensitive to the light in the yellow part of the spectrum (close to the center of visible light). In addition, different parts of the eye absorb or transmit different wavelengths of light as well. For example, the cornea and lens will absorb (block out) ultraviolet light but allow blue light, which is slightly less intense to pass through. Now, this blue light is the light that has the highest level of energy to reach the retina. It is important to realize this since the central part of the retina (the macula) is constantly stimulated with this light when we are awake. It is for this reason that our eyes "filter" out some of this blue light. The pigment accumulates in the macula to help reduce glare and strain on the retina.

The blue-light issue had not been significant until the development of the tablet computer, which uses light emitting diode (LED) technology to generate images. The light from LED bulbs has more blue light than traditional incandescent bulbs or fluorescent bulbs. Some research has associated blue light with negative effects on the eyes in a few ways.

Blue light stimulates the reduction of melatonin in the body. The pineal gland produces melatonin, a hormone that is responsible for a person's circadian rhythm, or wakefulness. It controls our biological clocks and allows us to wake up in the mornings and sleep at night. Light levels that enter the eye will increase or decrease melatonin production, allowing us to go to sleep or wake up. One way to remember this is to think of the blue sky in the morning, which will allow us to wake up. If you are exposed to too much blue light at night (as you would be by using a tablet, laptop, or smartphone before bed), there will be a decrease in your level of melatonin at precisely the time at which you require the hormone, making it difficult for you to fall asleep.

Another issue with blue light is that it focuses in a different place than its opposite color, red light. Being a higher energy of light, blue light scatters more (another reason the sky is blue) and can focus in front of the retina, whereas red light will focus behind the retina. This issue is chromatic aberration. Too much blue light, unfortunately, can cause the eye to strain, as if it were nearsighted.

Lastly, excessive blue-light exposure has been considered a possible causative factor in age-related macular degeneration (AMD). While it is true that it is the highest energy of light reaching the retina, and the macula in particular, there are no studies that confirm the idea that excessive blue-light exposure can cause AMD. In addition, the amount of blue light coming from a display screen is minimal compared the blue light that comes from sunlight. You would have to spend fifteen hours looking at a computer to get the same amount of blue-light exposure you would experience by being outside in the sun for just one hour. Therefore, this issue has proven not to be much of a concern for the many scientists who have studied it.

CONCLUSION

We live our lives in a bright and colorful world. Yet we experience eyestrain in a variety of viewing conditions. The eyes can adapt themselves to many viewing conditions, but they can fall prey to overuse or awkward viewing situations that we create in our modern world. It is important to be cautious regarding how we use our eyes because they are irreplaceable. In the next chapter, we will discuss the various types of eyestrain we may encounter and how we can reduce their effects.

7

Visual Stress

In the previous chapters, we addressed many of the sources of eye-strain, ranging from computer viewing to paper reading and delays in vision development. There is a fine line between "stress" and "strain," however, so now we should broaden our view of how stress affects our body. Whether stress is physical or mental, it is something that we deal with every day of our lives, and it can manifest in a number of different forms and conditions.

DEFINING STRESS

Stress is an organism's response to a stressor, which may be internal or external to the organism. Stress is the body's method of reacting to a condition such as a threat, challenge, or physical barrier. Stress can be physical or psychological. The body reacts automatically to stress, using the autonomic nervous system and through the secretion of hormones typically produced by the adrenal glands. Physical stress, when it becomes chronic, can lead to strain on any or all organ systems, including the eyes.

Everyone experiences stress differently, and that which stresses you out may not even bother someone else, and vice versa. Still, most human beings will likely react the same to stressors. This is because the stress response is your body's way of dealing with tough or demanding situations. For example, stress can make your heart beat faster, make you breathe rapidly, make you sweat, and make you tense up. It can also give you a burst of energy. Unfortunately, it can have a negative effect on your eyes and your sight.

Visual Stress

Because we use our eyes every waking moment of every day, they are constantly taking in light, transforming that light into nerve impulses, interacting with the brain to help control our body movements, and all the while continuing to move around to scan the horizon or to read written materials. It is actually amazing that eyestrain is not more commonly experienced, but since our vision is so critical to our survival, nature has provided us with a great deal of flexibility, through which the eyes can adapt.

Visual stress is a perceptual processing condition that can cause reading difficulties, headaches, and visual problems from exposure to patterns in text. Visual stress can be linked to dyslexia and similar visual learning difficulties. Sufferers might experience print distortion and fatigue when reading. Other possible symptoms might include movement of the printed text, blurring of print, letters changing size or shape, patterns in the print, halos of color surrounding words, and tiring easily while reading. This type of stress is a condition that can directly lead to eyestrain.

The visual system (which consists of the eyes, optic nerves, and visual perception in the brain) is our main interaction with the world. We too often expect our eyes to function normally during the early growth years, but some bodies (and eyes) react differently to stress than others. Eyecare practitioners can test the abilities of the eyes to ensure they are functioning with optimum efficiency and, if they are not, make recommendations on how to rebalance the visual system to allow the eyes to be used without experiencing strain.

SOURCES OF VISUAL STRESS

So, what are some of these areas of eyestrain that can stress the visual system to malfunction? Many times, it is a matter of eye coordination. Given that we have two eyes that must coordinate their focusing and eye movements together to maintain single binocular vision, the muscle systems of the eyes must react normally without excessive stress.

Muscle Stress

As we discussed earlier, the two muscle systems of the eyes must match up to move the eyes in conjunction with each other. The muscles on the outside of the eyes, called striated muscles, turn the eyes from side to side and up and down in all directions. Each muscle that performs this movement is about 200 times stronger than is required to move the eyeball in any particular direction. Thus, it is rare that a weakened muscle causes a "turned" eye.

The muscles within the eye, called smooth muscles, are responsible for the focusing mechanism to allow light from different distances to focus onto the retina. These muscles control the crystalline lens and allow for clear vision at all distances. If these two muscles systems are not in absolute coordination with each other, visual stress develops. This is the only place in the body that both of these two muscle systems must work together.

Visual discomfort is a response to this misalignment. These two muscles systems, if struggling to coordinate with each other, will force one or the other system to adapt, which can result in conditions such as nearsightedness, a particular form of dyslexia, under achievement, or, of course, eyestrain.

It can also happen that the eyes, when working under normal viewing conditions, react normally. Yet this system might break down if the same eyes are used in a situation of extreme demand, such as writing a book or straining to see under less than optimal viewing conditions. One example would be putting the normal functioning visual system in a condition of viewing a poor quality image on a computer screen. The poor image could result in the focusing muscles being forced to attempt to clear the image continually but never being successful in this task. This problem could eventually lead to any number of different symptoms of eyestrain.

Overload Demand

This brings up the concept of workload. We often think of eyestrain as a result of a problem with the visual system, but sometimes it is simply a matter of demanding too much of our own eyes. Think of a long-distance truck driver who drives daily on highways for many hours in a row. This person might be able to handle the "visual load" very well, moving the eyes from the highway to the mirrors to the gauges back to the highway and so on for hours at a time. Aside from conventional late-night fatigue, their eyes might handle the job very well. Now, think of that same person sitting in front of a computer for eight straight hours. Would they be able to handle that type of visual demand? Not necessarily. Thus, it is a balance between the viewing situations and the abilities of the visual system that determines whether someone experiences visual stress or eyestrain.

Another visual demand that might be more common today is meeting deadlines. Whether it is a student finishing a term paper or a newspaper reporter getting the scoop for the next edition, the stress of a deadline can affect all functional aspects of a person's performance of a task. The expression of this form of psychological stress may occur as eye pain, headaches, digestive upset, or many other forms of strain on the body.

Glare

We briefly covered the topic of glare in Chapter 3. (See page 26.) There are two general categories of glare: discomfort glare and disability glare. Each of these has the potential to generate visual stress and eyestrain. In addition, there are two instances of glare: direct and indirect glare. One cause of glare can be a strong contrast in brightness between different objects in your field of vision.

Discomfort glare will cause you to want to look away from an object that is overly illuminated. Think of the glare of oncoming headlights while driving at night. Disability glare can impair the ability to view objects without necessarily causing discomfort. Light scatter within the eyeball leads to disability glare, as it reduces the contrast between the object being viewed and the surrounding area.

Recall that the retina of the eye has rods and cones, which are receptors of light. The cones are responsible for daytime vision and color perception, whereas the rods respond to nighttime vision and contrast between black and white. One might think of humans as having two retinas—one for day vision and one for night vision. You can experience the transition between the two retinas by walking into a darkened movie theater on a bright day. At first, the entire theater might look completely black because your "daytime" retina is still at work while looking at a dark field of view. Once you have been inside for a few seconds, objects in the darkened theater become visible as the rods start to take over the "nighttime" viewing task.

This is why one should have more uniform luminance in the field of view. High-contrast situations, such as a bright computer display in a dark room, cause an imbalance between the "two retinas," leading them to compete with each other for dominance. A more unified luminous field of view will be more relaxing for the eyes and reduce the likelihood of eyestrain.

One of the main instances of glare occurs in night driving, which is also one of the most difficult tasks we perform with our eyes. There are a number of factors that make night driving a challenge, even for the people who have excellent vision at all other times.

First, let us consider the anatomy of the retina. As we discussed in Chapter 1, there are rods and cones in the retina. The macula, where we have our sharpest vision, consists of only cones, with no rods at all. The more central areas of the retina have more cones and the more peripheral areas have an increasingly number of rods. Thus, when we view nighttime objects, we are not using our most central and most sensitive retinal cells.

Next, consider the scattering of light, which can lead to glare. In general, glare decreases our ability to see objects more clearly. Headlights from oncoming cars can create a glare situation that is difficult to overcome and decreases our visual ability. In addition, if someone is an older driver (typically late sixties or older), there is a possibility of cataracts. A cataract in the crystalline lens within the eye will lead to a loss of transparency, which causes light to scatter, thereby decreasing contrast and clarity.

The visual system is designed to see most clearly during the day and to sleep at night. Our modern society, however, has put other demands on the visual system, and we must try to adapt. One of the side effects of this adaptation is eyestrain.

Contrast Sensitivity

Contrast is comparing one item with another. It is also important in being able to recognize one item standing out from another, such as writing on paper or letters on a computer screen. The retina is "wired" to tune in to the contrast between objects so that we can distinguish them from each other more clearly. This is known as contrast sensitivity.

When there is not enough contrast between objects, they become less visible. When this occurs, our eyes can strain to attempt to make out the image clearly. Since we focus on objects in our field of view, these objects need to stand out from the background of our view. Think of viewing a mountain scene on a clear day as opposed to one where there is fog or haze in the atmosphere. Light scatters in the haze and thus we lose much of the contrast of the mountains in our view. This is also important in how easily we read text on paper or see other cars while driving at night. Therefore, having good contrast sensitivity is important in maintaining clear and comfortable vision.

Headaches

The most common complaint among eyecare patients is headache. It is very often the first sign of a vision-related problem. Almost everyone, though, experiences headache at one time or another. Common causes include stress, tension, anxiety, allergies, constipation, coffee consumption, hunger, sinus pressure, muscular tension, hormone imbalance, trauma, nutritional deficiency, alcohol consumption, drug use, smoking, fever, and, yes, eyestrain. Experts estimate that about 90 percent of all headaches are tension headaches, and 6 percent are migraines. Tension headaches, as the name implies, are related to muscular tension. Migraines result from, most likely, a disturbance in the blood circulation to the brain. Another relatively common type of headache is the cluster headache. This severe, recurrent headache strikes about 1 million Americans each year.

Vision-related headaches most often are located toward the front of the head, although there are a few exceptions. They occur most often at the middle or end of the day, are not present upon waking in the morning, and do not produce visual auras such as flashing lights. These headaches often strike in a different pattern on weekends than they do during the week, or do not occur at all on weekends. They also affect one side of the head more than they do the other, and symptoms that are more general may accompany them.

Because of all the symptoms that accompany headaches, it is important that your doctor obtain a thorough history from you to determine the type of headaches from which you suffer. You should be aware of the time of the headache's onset, specific location of the pain, frequency, duration, severity, and precipitating factors, such as stress, certain foods, or medications. You should also note such associated signs and symptoms as nausea, vomiting, light sensitivity, and sound sensitivity.

It is important to discuss more thoroughly the subject of migraines, since they are associated with numerous eye symptoms. The migraine headache is a disorder consisting of localized symptoms that may or may not actually be associated with headaches. The eye symptoms are similar to those of many other diseases, so you should seek professional care in order to properly diagnose and treat the disorder. Migraines have a number of phases that exhibit definite symptoms. The first phase is the *prodromal*, or *premonitory*, phase, during which you might suffer irritability, depression, light sensitivity, or sound sensitivity. These symptoms may show up as early as two days before the actual headache. The second phase is the *aura* phase, which consists of visual symptoms such as flashing lights, halos around lights, zigzagging of lines, and distortion of shapes and colors. This phase typically evolves over twenty minutes and is commonly but not always followed by a headache. The headache may throb, be located on one or both sides of the head, and last from four to seventy-two hours. The final phase is called the *postdromal* phase, which can leave you feeling washed out and exhausted. Because migraine headaches have a visual aspect to them, eye doctors are often the first health practitioner consulted in the matter.

To summarize, possible visual effects of migraines include but are not limited to the following: light sensitivity, blurred vision, aura, blind spots, flashes of colored lights, and tunnel vision. Any of these symptoms may have a variety of causes and should be discussed with an eyecare professional.

Long-Term Effects

So, what may be the long-term effects of eyestrain on the eyes and visual system in general? Well, people make three likely adjustments when they push the limits of stress on their bodies. They adapt, reject, or absorb.

If you are subject to eyestrain on a regular basis, your body will try to achieve a state of equilibrium, which means it will attempt to adapt itself to reduce the level of stress. Where the eyes are concerned, this involves the process of accommodation, or focusing on a near-viewing object. When the eyes look anywhere within twenty feet, the crystalline lens inside the eye must "thicken" to increase the focal power of the eye so that near objects can become clear. There are muscles that surround this lens that contract to allow this thickening to occur. As previously mentioned, these muscles are called ciliary muscles, which are the type of smooth muscle that can contract for long periods without tiring and are controlled by the (involuntary) autonomic nervous system. While the image of this near-viewing object is clear, these muscles must maintain their contraction for the entire time you are reading, sewing, or doing any near-viewing task.

This process also places strain on the internal parts of the eye and increases the pressure within the eye. Combine these conditions with poor lighting and the stress within the eye can cause the eye to elongate. This allows the image of a near object to fall on the retina with less effort. When this situation occurs on a regular basis, the eye will elongate permanently to allow for easier near viewing. While near viewing is now performed with less stress, distance vision is now out of focus. This person has "adapted" to their near-viewing stress and is now nearsighted.

Quite often an eye exam will reveal this nearsighted condition and some doctors will simply prescribe glasses to make distance viewing clear once again. The patient, however, will continue using his or her eyes "incorrectly" and continue down the path of nearsightedness, possibly getting stronger glasses every year or so.

If the near-viewing stress continues and the visual system cannot adapt to this environment, the person may simply "reject" the stress and quit reading or doing any significant amount of close-viewing tasks. This is common with juvenile delinquents who shun any reading tasks and are labeled as "poor readers." There may be other conditions contributing to this rejection, but very often, visual stress is involved on some level.

In an ideal situation, the visual system will be able to absorb this stress and bounce back the next day to function normally again. This resilience requires a robust visual system (in which the muscles coordinate properly), optimal lighting, a viewing distance that is not too close, taking breaks from near viewing, optimal nutrition, and other factors.

CONCLUSION

As you now know, stress can affect the visual system in many ways, and most will lead to one form of eyestrain or another. Eyestrain is a common complaint from patients, but it is a challenge for doctors to confirm the cause of the condition without more follow-up details. With the information discussed here, you should now be able to offer more detailed information to your doctor, which may be of assistance in resolving your eyestrain.

Aging

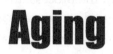

The process of aging certainly affects all your all body parts, but aside from some of the aches and pains of getting older, you are only as old as you think you are—or as young. So, with this idea in mind, what can you do to limit eyestrain as you age? This chapter covers some of the challenges we face as we age and still try to use our eyes with ease and clarity.

During the first forty years of life, our bodies typically perform all our normal functions well. They grow to their maximum size, they turn food into its basic nutrients to carry on our life functions, and they become able produce the next generation of offspring. There comes a time, however, when various aspects of our bodies begin to slow down and, in some cases, wear out. This is the nature of life, but the fact is that there is much more to the process of aging.

Consider the fact that the first *Homo sapiens* lived to be, on average, approximately twenty-five to thirty years old, and that the average American life span in 1900 was only about forty-seven years old. This average is now closing in on eighty years old. Yes, a lot has to do with the fact that we have conquered most infectious diseases, but problems arise when lifestyle-based diseases, such as hypertension, diabetes, heart problems, and many more, complicate life span. It has been said that humans now have a longer life span but a shorter "health span." In fact, the typical American is in a state of disease for an average of seven years prior to death. We may be living longer lives but not necessarily better lives. Unfortunately, too many of us hand over our health needs to doctors without taking responsibility for our own health, which includes the state of our eye health.

We use our eyes every waking moment of every day, so they are prone to stress more as we age. While eyestrain can occur at any age, three factors are involved in the process: the physical state of our eyes, our viewing environments, and our visual habits. Let us review some of these conditions to see how age can lead to strain on our eyes.

THE STATE OF YOUR EYES

We have covered many of the possible optical conditions of the eyes that might affect the way we see, namely nearsightedness, farsightedness, and astigmatism. Each of these conditions can adversely affect the way we see things and how much strain our visual system experiences as we age.

Nearsightedness

One who is nearsighted has clear vision at close viewing distances. If one who is nearsighted looks at a near object, such as a book, computer display, or any other task within arm's length, then the object is seen clearly and little strain is experienced. When a nearsighted person views distant objects, however, they experience a blurred image and attempt to clear the view by squinting or straining their eyes.

The development of nearsightedness has traditionally been an issue of early life. It is rare for someone to be born with nearsighted eyes; the process typically begins in early school years (ages eight through ten) and tends to continue gradually until the late teenage years (eighteen or nineteen). With the increased use of digital displays, however, nearsightedness seems to be showing up as late as the early twenties and continuing into the early thirties.

As the eyes age and lose their ability to focus (a condition known as presbyopia, which is discussed on page 84), nearsighted people actually have an advantage, due to their ability to see clearly up close without the use of corrective lenses. When most people over forty are putting on glasses to read, the nearsighted person just takes theirs off. Now, this result will depend on how much nearsightedness the person exhibits, as well as the viewing distance of the near-viewing object. For example, if someone is moderately nearsighted and attempts to view a book at sixteen inches away (normal reading distance), the text might be in perfect focus with no additional effort required. Threading a needle, though, might be a bit more difficult a task for this person to accomplish.

Farsightedness

Most newborns are a bit farsighted. In an ideal situation, this farsightedness decreases gradually over the first few years of life and, hopefully, settles into a state of emmetropia, which refers to a state of clear distance vision with no effort. In a farsighted condition, the person has to actively focus the eyes just to view a distant object clearly, which typically can be accomplished if the person is young enough (usually under forty years of age) and has enough focusing ability. To see clearly up close, though, a person must perform the standard amount of focusing of the eyes in addition to the focusing required for clear distance vision. Thus, a farsighted person is tasked with possibly two or three times the amount of focusing as a person with "normal" eyesight might do. This is a very stressful condition, and is often the leading cause of eyestrain.

Since the eye gradually loses its ability to focus as we age, a farsighted person might actually notice difficulty with near-viewing objects earlier than a non-farsighted forty-year-old might. Studies show that the maximum focusing ability of the eye is reached at about the age of ten and continually decreases as we age. For viewing a near object comfortably at about sixteen inches away, the eye requires about five units of focusing. This point occurs at about forty-two years of age. In order to see near objects clearly, a farsighted forty-plus individual will have to move reading material further away in order to see it clearly.

Astigmatism

Astigmatism adds another complicating factor to the eyestrain issue. With astigmatism, images coming into the eye are distorted, usually due to the uneven curvature of the cornea, and there is no point of focus of the light onto the retina. The eye might attempt to find the clearest point of focus, but will continually have to focus the lens within the eye to find this "sweet spot," and there is no guarantee that this point even exists. This continual focusing is a common source of eyestrain and creates a blurred image both at distance and near viewing. As noted earlier, the loss of focusing ability with age makes this extra focusing a significant challenge, and one that can lead to significant eyestrain.

Presbyopia

As recently stated, maximum focusing ability occurs at about the age of ten years old, at which point most children can focus on objects located almost to the tip of the noses. At the age of fifteen, it recedes to a point about three inches away from the eyes. At twenty years old, the focusing limit is about six inches away. At twenty-five years old, it is around twelve inches away, and at thirty years old, it is another few inches farther. At this point, we start considering the comfortable focusing ability as opposed to the previously mentioned maximum. The fact is that we might have a decent maximum ability to focus but cannot maintain that effort for any length of time. This is the reason for eyestrain—we typically should use only about half our maximum ability to read comfortably.

Around the age of forty, the eyes can easily focus at a sixteen-inch reading distance but may have difficulty maintaining that focus for an extended period. In the next few years, the forty-five year old will have to adjust reading distance, extending it to around an arm's length away. By fifty years old, the average person cannot clear the image on a near object without glasses. All this, of course, depends on the condition of the eyes (if one eye is nearsighted, you can just remove your glasses and see clearly up close). This loss of focusing ability with age is called *presbyopia* (prez-bee-OH-pee-ah) and comes from the Greek *presbys*, meaning old, and *opia*, meaning vision. It is a part of the normal aging process and happens to everyone.

HOW THESE CONDITIONS AFFECT EYESTRAIN

The above conditions can occur in one eye or both, but regardless of each eye's condition both eyes must coordinate with each other to assure single, binocular vision (seeing with both eyes). This is the main state that allows us to judge distances and maintain true stereoscopic vision. One might be able to learn how to judge distances with only one functional eye, but the experience is much different with the involvement of two eyes.

When viewing near objects, our eyes perform two actions: accommodation, which refers to an increase in the power of the crystalline lens within the eye, and convergence, which refers to a turning in of the line of sight of each eye. The process of accommodation maintains the clarity of an object, while the convergence process aims the eyes correctly so that both eyes remain fixated on an object. These two systems are neurologically connected so that they work in unison. Therefore, when you focus on a close object, the eyes automatically turn in, and when the eyes turn in, the lenses increase in focal power to maintain a clear focus. With presbyopia, however, you lose the ability to focus the crystalline lens. Thus, when you view a close object, you must turn your eyes in toward the object without the help of accommodation. This process is more difficult and can lead to eyestrain, most typically with the symptom of "tired" eyes.

So, can you delay presbyopia? It is unlikely that you will be the only person who does not ever lose focusing ability with age, but there is something you could do as a work-around in the process. There is a vision relaxation technique known as accommodative rock (see page 145), in which you alternately focus up close and then far away. This technique forces and then relaxes the crystalline lens in the eye. As we age, this lens tends to thicken, as previously described, but at least you will be able to keep as much flexibility in the lens as possible for as long as possible. Just make sure to do this technique at least two or three times a day before you start to notice a loss of near focusing. It's easier to prevent a loss of vision than to try to recover it.

THE VIEWING ENVIRONMENT

If you work in an office or at home, most likely your work will involve looking at a computer's display monitor. Every occupation has its own visual demands. Most offices have uniform illumination to cover all areas of the office evenly. This was an acceptable environment when viewing paper-based forms and documents, which require reflected light to view their texts easily. With today's computer-based offices, however, uniform lighting can lead to eyestrain. The same thing holds true if you are working at home. Few home offices are set up with the proper lighting to accommodate a computer screen.

Task lighting, usually in the form of a desk lamp, is the optimum way to view a paper copy while still having a dimmer ambient light for the optimum viewing of a computer screen. Normally, computer displays create an image by using backlighting; they do not require reflected light to see the images. It is generally recommended that the brightness of a computer display be approximately equal to the immediate surrounding illumination. Therefore, if you maintain a light background on the display, then the room lighting around the monitor should be somewhat lighter than it would be if you had a darker display background. Conversely, if you maintain a darker background on the screen, the immediate surrounding brightness in the room could be dimmer.

As you learned in Chapter 6, your parents were right when they said, "Don't watch TV in the dark." The higher contrast between a brightly lit computer display and a completely darkened room is too much for the retina to comfortably process. In addition, this issue gets worse as the eyes age because we get more scattering of light—most typically due to the lens losing some of its transparency—which reduces our ability to distinguish contrast. The loss of contrast leads to age-related eyestrain.

Now, reading a book is much different due to a few factors. First, the book tends to be positioned in a lower viewing angle, on either a desk or lap. This is the preferred position since the lines of sight between the two eyes not only converge toward each other but also do so at a lower viewing angle. Thus, a lower viewing angle is less stressful on the eyes.

Secondly, a book requires reflected light and is typically in better balance with overall room illumination. The uniformity in lighting is much less stressful on the retina, which can more easily focus on the letters in the book. This brings up a third factor, which is the contrast between the letters and the background of the book. This high contrast—black letters on white paper—causes the letters to stand out more, making the text easier to read and less likely to cause eyestrain.

YOUR VISUAL HABITS

How you use your eyes and your visual abilities will dictate the level of eyestrain you may feel, and these abilities change as you age. When you look at near objects, you activate your eye muscles to accommodate your eyes to the near-viewing task. Contrary to popular folklore, the eye muscles do not actually weaken with age. This near-point viewing becomes more challenging with age because the lens loses its flexibility. Recall that the crystalline lens within the eye flexes to change shape to allow it to increase the focusing power of the eye. The lens, however, continues to grow as you age, becoming thicker and thicker every year. Given the limited space within the eye itself, it is impossible to maintain a maximum expansion of the lens thickness when the lens in a relaxed state is thicker than it used to be.

Visually speaking, when something is farther away, it requires less effort on the focusing system of our eyes. For example, occupations such as truck driving, forest ranger, law enforcement, and firefighting might seem to fit this model, since most of their viewing is at a far distance. (Let us, for a moment, not consider the report writing that many occupations require.) This far-distance viewing is less stressful on the focusing muscles within the eyes and is therefore "low stress." A young person who has clear lenses inside the eyes and is not bothered by bright lights might not notice much eyestrain. A cataract, however, (even an early one), which is a clouding of the lens and typically occurs with advanced age, will cause light to scatter, reducing contrast and making objects harder to see. The eyes will strain to see, sometimes calling in the forehead and eyelid muscles to help, but this compensatory action will cause even more strain.

When viewing near objects for extended periods, our focusing muscles tense up for the entire viewing period and will likely experience more stress and, eventually, eyestrain. Occupations in this category are more office-based, such as administrative assistant, customer service, computer programmer, dentist, engineer, and many more. These occupations require continual focusing of the eyes to see clearly and are more likely to cause eyestrain. This type of worker will experience these kinds of issues earlier and more severely because of the loss of ability to focus. Due to the loss of focusing ability with age, an older worker may experience these symptoms more significantly.

Another situation is when the eyes must be continually adjusted to see far and then near, and then far again. This situation is more common in sports that involve an object continually changing its distance from the viewer. For example, a tennis player must be able to keep the ball in sight as it travels about 150 miles per hour toward them, and to see where it lands when it is returned to the opponent's side of the court. These actions require constant adjustment of the focusing muscles as well as the eye muscles on the outside of the eyeball, moving both eyes in unison to track the ball. This constant adjustment requires more effort in the aging eye, due to the slower response in focusing.

EYESTRAIN IN RETIREMENT

You might think that once someone retires from the workforce, his or her visual strain is not an issue anymore. I used to think this true as well, until I saw a patient who had recently retired from a long career as an accountant. I suggested that since he was now retired, he might not have to worry as much about the amount of time spent in front of his computer. His response was, "But doc, I'm playing video games all day long." So much for that concept!

Today, when retirees stop working at their daylong occupations, many have time to do more recreational activities, which may include sewing, reading, card games, model building, and, yes, playing video games—all near-viewing tasks. While most retirees will likely wear glasses for reading (or take off their glasses to read if they are near-sighted), it is still common for them to experience eyestrain if not enough light is available for their viewing tasks.

Aging changes the structures within the eye, creating new lighting requirements. A sixty-year-old person requires three times more light than a twenty-year-old person for proper viewing. The crystalline lens within the eye gradually begins to turn from clear to a slight brownish

Keep Reading

If you enjoy reading, it is important to find ways to continue taking part in this pastime. You do not need to give it up. Here are four things you can do to make reading easier.

1. **Improve Your Lighting.** By simply getting a brighter light or chang-ing the type of light you use, you can make a big difference in your reading comfort. Less magnification is needed when proper lighting is available. Use brighter bulbs and lamps that can be adjusted so that the light is directed onto your reading material. Use a lamp that has not only adjustable height but also pivot points to direct the light onto your book page.

2. **Read Large-Print Books.** You can purchase just about any book you want in large print. Not only do large-print books have larger fonts, but they also have better contrast and allow for more blank space.

color, thereby decreasing the amount of light traveling through the eye. This is a common issue of aging and becomes more significant if a cataract develops in the lens, which is a loss of transparency within the crystalline lens, the chances of which gradually increase with age. By the age of eighty, over 90 percent of the population has a cataract, which is why cataract surgery is the most common surgery performed in the United States.

So, how do we address some of these issues? The first thing to do is adjust the lighting to maximize visibility. As the lens yellows, more light is required. Secondly, try to increase the size of the print of that which you are reading. The advantage of using digital displays is that the print size can be easily increased with a touch of a button, rather than having to purchase large-print books. Of course, if reading becomes a significant issue, audiobooks offer an additional option to overcome failing eyesight.

Virtual Assistants

A virtual assistant is a software program that can perform tasks or services for an individual, usually just using voice commands. As of 2017,

Some books are printed on special paper that has no glare. Your local library should carry a large selection of books in large print.

3. **Use an E-Reader.** Most books in print are now available as e-books—in other words, as books that can be read on a digital device. The unique feature of e-books is that the reader can increase the size of the font on a page to a size that allows for comfortable reading. Often the reader can also adjust the device's background lighting to be brighter or softer, which is helpful, as sometimes the wrong background lighting on a digital screen causes eyestrain.

4. **Try Audio Books.** While audio books have been around for a long time, the trend to listen to recorded titles has exploded in recent years. The beauty of listening to books instead of reading them allows the eyes to rest. And while some people find comfort in reading a physical book, occasionally listening to a book can be comforting in its own way, while also preventing eyestrain.

the capabilities and usage of virtual assistants are expanding rapidly, with new products entering the market. The most widely used assistants in the United States are Apple's Siri, Google's Assistant, Amazon's Alexa, and Samsung's Bixby. Virtual assistants work via text (online chat), voice commands, or by taking or uploading images.

You might be able to simplify your life using voice commands or voice activation. This type of technology is a cloud-based voice service that is always getting smarter and adding new skills. If you would like better sound connect for this voice technology, use a smart speaker or connect your smart phone to an external speaker via Bluetooth or with the help of an audio cable.

This virtual assistant technology benefits those with vision problems. They are made to facilitate common tasks for you. With a simple voice command, you can check the weather, play music, set an alarm, set a timer, ask a question, manage your calendar, and more. For instance, if you want to know what time it is, check your local weather, or just listen to your favorite tunes, all you have to do is ask. There is no need to check large-number clocks, search online for your local weather, or write down a reminder to get eggs.

You can set up this technology for use in many different rooms of your home. In your kitchen, you can ask Alexa to play your favorite music or make a shopping list. In your bedroom, you can ask Siri to set an alarm or play sleep-promoting music. You can also connect them to smart-home devices such as lights, thermostat, garage door and sprinklers. To activate the unit, you simply use the unit's initiation word and then give it a command or ask it a question.

As with any technology, these services are always getting smarter, with new skills and updates constantly incorporated into their programs. Check the Resources (page 167) for more information on these assistants.

Traditional Reading Magnifiers

Lighting and magnification are the two most important reading aids in helping you to see words clearly. While the world of digital screens may provide a means of increasing word size and controlling lighting, the fact is that many magazines, newspapers, bills, documents, and letters require magnifying devices to be read. When people talk about making sure to read "the fine print," for many, this task cannot be done without a magnifier. Most people prefer having a large area of print magnified rather than just a few words or just part of a sentence. Ideally, a full-page magnifier is the best for reading, depending on how much magnification a person needs.

Bigger, though, is not always better. A larger magnifier, such as a full-page magnifier, is also generally a weaker magnifier. This fact means that you will not find a full-page version that offers five-times magnification. Most full-page magnifiers offer only two-times magnification, making the print appear two times its original size. If a magnifier also provides good lighting, however, the need for higher magnification may not be necessary.

A small magnifier, such as a handheld magnifying glass, offers more powerful magnification. If you need more than two-times magnification, then a smaller magnifier should help. A small handheld magnifier, which offers more power, such as a five-times magnifier, may help by making the words appear clearer and crisper, but the trade-off is less print will be visible. It can also be very tedious to hold a magnifier for any length of time in excess of that which you might spend on simple spot reading.

Magnifiers come in many styles and are often inexpensive. There are small dome magnifiers to glide over newsprint, floor-standing magnifiers to keep near your favorite reading chair, and many other types. You may want to have a couple of different reading magnifiers for different reading material. Sometimes you simply need to try a couple of reading magnifiers to find the ones that work best for you.

CONCLUSION

Everyone gets older, but the pace of aging is dependent on many, many variables. While we get our "blueprint" for our lifetimes from our genes, our environments play an important role in our rate of aging. It is unlikely that we would completely wear out our eyes by doing visually intensive work, but taking care of them is a lifelong process. Part of this process is feeding them well, thus the next chapter will explore how diet and nutrient intake can affect not only the structures of the eyeball but also the full functioning of the entire visual system.

9

Nutrition and Your Eyes

E very organ in the body relies on adequate nutrition to function properly. Your eyes are certainly no exception. You might be surprised to find out that the brain and visual system, while comprising only about 2 percent of your body weight, use up about 25 percent of your nutritional intake. Yes, this sounds like a lot, but there is a good reason for this level of need. The brain and eyes expend the most energy of all cells, so they need the most nutritional support in order to function optimally. This chapter discusses the nutrition your eyes—and your body—need for peak performance. It gives an overview of nutrition, explaining how it works and how it generally affects the body. In addition, it talks about macronutrients—water, carbohydrates, protein, and fats—and some selected micronutrients—vitamins and minerals—that are especially important to vision, and how all these nutrients may relate to eyestrain.

MACRONUTRIENTS

Macronutrients refer to any substances of which the body needs large amounts to survive. They are the essential ingredients to the building blocks of nutrition. They include water, carbohydrates, protein, and fat, all of which are required for the process of metabolism—the conversion of food into useable nutrients. Although macronutrients are critical for life itself, there are no federal guidelines regarding their intake, such as there are for vitamins and minerals. All macronutrients are required to some degree and available in the foods we eat. Let us review macronutrients and see how they interact with our bodies to supply the fuel for life.

Water

Water is an essential nutrient that is involved in every function of the body. It helps to transport other nutrients and waste products in and out of cells. It is necessary for all of the digestive, absorptive, circulatory, and excretory functions of the body, as well as for the body's utilization of water-soluble vitamins. It is also needed for the maintenance of proper body temperature. The human body, like our planet itself, is, in fact, two-thirds water.

Replenishing your body's supply of water, which is continually drained through sweating and elimination, is very important. To keep your body functioning properly, you must drink approximately eight 8-ounce glasses of water each day. While the body can survive without food for about five weeks, it cannot survive without water for more than about five days. The body's initial response to a loss of fluid is to preserve the amount of fluid still in the body by conserving water. This leads to various symptoms of dehydration, including thirst, dry mouth, decreased urine output, muscle cramps, headache, lightheadedness, sleepiness, and a lack of tear production. When the eyes stop producing tears, they are no longer properly lubricated, which can lead to dry eye, eyestrain, and vision problems.

Carbohydrates

Carbohydrates supply the body with the energy it needs to function. They are found almost exclusively in fruit, some root vegetables, cereals, honey, and dairy milk. Of course, processed foods also tend to contain a significant amount of carbohydrates.

Carbohydrates are generally divided into two groups: simple and complex. Simple carbohydrates are categorized as such because they contain simple sugars, which include fructose and glucose (found in fruit), and lactose (found in milk produced by lactation). Fruit is one of the richest natural sources of simple carbohydrates. Complex carbohydrates are also made up of sugars, but these sugar molecules are strung together into longer, more complex chains. Sources of complex carbohydrates include whole wheat and whole grain, as well as starchy foods such as potatoes.

Carbohydrates are the main source of blood glucose, which is a major fuel for all of the body's cells, and the main source of energy for the brain and red blood cells. Except for fiber, which cannot be digested, both simple and complex carbohydrates are converted into glucose. The glucose is then either used directly to provide energy for the body, or stored in the liver for future use. When a person consumes more calories than the body needs, a portion of the carbohydrates consumed may also be stored in the body as fat. Thus, when too many carbohydrates are consumed or not processed properly, excess fatty tissue accumulates and stresses the body. There are actually no carbohydrates stored in the body; they are just used to produce energy for the body to function. Given the level of energy production in the retina and eye muscles, complex carbohydrates are critical to keep eyes functioning at an optimum level on a daily basis.

Protein

Protein is essential for growth and development. It provides the body with energy, and the body uses it for the manufacture of hormones, antibodies, enzymes, and tissues. It also helps to maintain the proper acid-alkaline balance in the body. When you consume protein, it is broken down in the body into amino acids, which are the building blocks of protein. Some amino acids are classified as nonessential. This does not mean that they are unnecessary, but rather that they do not have to come from the diet because they are manufactured by the body from other amino acids. The remaining amino acids are essential, meaning that they are not synthesized by the body and must be obtained from the diet.

Because of the importance of consuming proteins that provide all the essential amino acids, dietary proteins are divided into two groups according to the amino acids they contain. Complete proteins, which constitute the first group, contain ample amounts of all the essential amino acids. These proteins are found in meat, fish, poultry, cheese, eggs, and milk. Incomplete proteins, which constitute the second group, contain only some of the essential amino acids. These proteins are found in foods such as grains, legumes, and leafy green vegetables.

Although it is important to consume the full range of amino acids, both essential and nonessential, it is not necessary to get them from meat, fish, poultry, and the other complete-protein foods. In fact, because of their high fat content, most of these foods should be eaten in moderation. It is possible to create complete proteins by combining various incomplete-protein foods. This is called food combining. For instance, although beans and brown rice are both quite rich in protein, each lack one or more of the essential amino acids. When you combine beans and brown rice, however, or when you combine either one with any of a number of other protein-rich foods, you form a complete protein that is a high-quality substitute for meat.

The eyes and visual system depend on proteins as building blocks of structure. The white of the eye (sclera) is made up of collagen, which is formed from amino acids, just like protein. This provides a strong structure to keep the eye from becoming elongated and myopic. In addition, the crystalline lens in the eye is made up solely of proteins and requires continual nutrients from the aqueous fluid to maintain its clarity.

Fat

Although much attention has been focused on the need to reduce the amount of *fat* in the diet, the body does need some fat. During infancy and childhood, fat is necessary for normal brain development, since about 60 percent of the brain is made up of fat. Throughout life, it provides energy and supports growth. Fat is, in fact, the most concentrated source of energy available to the body. After the age of two, however, the body requires only small amounts of fat—much less than what is provided by the average American diet. What most people do not realize is that eating fat does not necessarily make you fat.

Fat is composed of building blocks called fatty acids. There are three major categories of fatty acids—saturated, polyunsaturated, and monounsaturated. Saturated fatty acids are found primarily in animal products, including dairy items, such as whole milk, cream, and cheese, and fatty meats such as beef, veal, lamb, pork, and ham. The fat marbling that you see in beef and pork is composed of saturated fat. Some vegetable products—including coconut oil, palm kernel, oil, and vegetable shortening—are also high in saturated fat. The liver uses saturated fat to manufacture cholesterol. Therefore, excessive dietary intake of saturated fat can significantly raise the blood-cholesterol level, especially the level of low-density lipoproteins (LDLs), or "bad" cholesterol.

Polyunsaturated fatty acids are found in the greatest abundance in corn, soybean, safflower, and sunflower oils. Certain fish oils are also high in the polyunsaturated fat. Unlike the saturated fat, the polyunsaturated fat may actually lower your total blood-cholesterol level. In doing so, however, they also have a tendency, when present in large amounts, to reduce your high-density lipoproteins (HDLs), or "good" cholesterol. For this reason, the guidelines state that your intake of polyunsaturated fat should not exceed 10 percent of your total caloric intake.

Monounsaturated fatty acids are found mostly in vegetable and nut oils, such as olive, peanut, and canola. This type of fat appears to reduce the LDL blood level without affecting the HDL level in any way. This positive impact upon LDL cholesterol, however, is relatively modest. Guidelines recommend that intake of monounsaturated fat be kept between 10 and 15 percent of total caloric intake.

Although most foods contain a combination of all three types of fatty acids, one of these types is usually predominant. Thus, a fat or oil is considered saturated or high in saturated fat when it comprises primarily saturated fatty acids. Saturated fat is usually solid at room temperature. A fat or oil composed mostly of polyunsaturated fatty acids is called polyunsaturated, while a fat or oil composed mostly of monounsaturated fatty acids is called monounsaturated.

Essential fatty acids (EFAs) get lots of attention in discussions on nutrition, but they are often misunderstood in connection to their effects on the eyes. The most widely discussed EFAs are omega-3 and omega-6 essential fatty acids. Omega-6 fatty acids are the most plentiful in our diet. They are in most everything we eat that contains fat, including meat, most seed oils, dairy products, and eggs. Excessive intake of omega-6s, however, can produce pro-inflammatory markers, which can lead to chronic inflammation. Omega-3 fatty acids are available in many seed oils and most all cold-water fatty fish. A proper balance of these fatty acids is essential to good overall and eye health. The daily intake recommendation of the Institute of Medicine is 4:1—four times as many omega-6 fatty acids as omega-3 fatty acids.

Fatty acids are stored in every cell membrane of your body. They have two primary functions. First, they ensure cellular fluidity, acting as gatekeepers for every cell and allowing vital nutrients to enter the cell and forcing destructive free radical debris out of the cells. Second, both omega-6 and omega-3 fatty acids can be converted into three different types of active molecules in a group known as prostaglandin E (PGE). Without going into extensive detail, prostaglandins achieve three processes: reduce inflammation and inhibit blood clotting (PGE1); constrict blood vessels, increase body temperature, and encourage blood clotting (PGE2); and play an important anti-inflammatory role (PGE3). All three of these prostaglandins are important for the body to maintain its health and balance.

Eicosapentaenoic acid (EPA) and docosahexaenoic acid (DHA) are two of the most discussed nutritional fatty acids. EPA is a polyunsaturated fatty acid (PUFA) that acts as a precursor for prostaglandin E3. The body converts alpha-linolenic acid (ALA) via a series of enzyme reactions into EPA. ALA is itself an essential fatty acid that the body needs from the diet. Food sources of ALA include flax seeds, pumpkin seeds, canola oil, soybeans, tofu, and walnuts. EPA is also a precursor to docosahexaenoic acid. Medical conditions such as diabetes and certain allergies, in addition to high cholesterol, aging, alcoholism, and nutritional deficiencies, may significantly limit the human body's capacity to convert ALA into EPA.

DHA, a long-chain omega-3 fatty acid, is found in tissues throughout the body, including the eye. It is a major structural and functional element of all membranes in the gray matter of the brain and the retina of the eye. It is also a key component of heart tissue. DHA is important for optimal brain and eye development in infants, and supports brain, eye, and cardiovascular health in adults. Adequate levels of DHA are important in learning and development in children. DHA is found in a limited selection of foods, including fatty fish and organ meats. The body can also synthesize DHA from its precursor alpha-linolenic acid, but the process is inefficient.

Some people recommend using flax oil as a stand-alone treatment for eye health because it contains a large amount of omega-3s and a small amount of omega-6s. Unfortunately, flax oil is highly unstable and contains none of the nutrient cofactors necessary to ensure the consistent conversion to either PGE1 or PGE3 anti-inflammatory prostaglandins, nor does it enhance the production of tear *lactoferrin*. Lactoferrin is another protein in tears that helps the eye to maintain a moist surface. It has antioxidant and antibacterial functions, and therefore promotes clear vision. The same can be said for any of the plant-based omega-3 fatty acids. In addition, the metabolism of medium-chain fatty acids (specifically ALA) into long-chain fatty acids (EPA/DHA) is very limited. Studies have shown that 10 percent or less of ALA will metabolize fully into EPA/DHA in women, and possibly only 1 percent or less in men.

Arachidonic acid (ARA), a long-chain omega-6 fatty acid, is the principal omega-6 in the brain, and it is abundant in other cells throughout the body. ARA is equally important for proper brain development in infants and is a precursor to a group of hormone-like substances called eicosanoids. Eicosanoids are important in immunity, blood clotting, and other vital functions in the body. Humans obtain ARA by eating foods such as meat, eggs, and milk. Both DHA and ARA fatty acids, along with lactoferrin, occur naturally in breast milk and support the mental and visual development of infants. The health benefits of DHA extend from prenatal development through adult life.

Your eyes require fat because they use fat-soluble vitamins, which are vitamins that must be dissolved by fat in order for the body to use them. Remember that the eyes are an extension of the brain, and DHA and EPA fats make up a large percentage of brain tissue. As mentioned earlier, DHA is essential for the growth and functional development of the brain in infants. DHA is also required to maintain normal brain functioning in adults. The inclusion of plentiful DHA in the diet improves learning ability, whereas deficiencies of DHA are associated with deficits in learning.

The Bottom Line

So, what is a good dietary balance of the macronutrients and how does it affect your eyes? Most experts agree that a good diet consists of about 2,000 calories a day for women, and about 2,500 calories a day for men. A proper balance of these calories consists of about 30 percent fat (mostly monounsaturated oils and only 7 percent of which should be saturated fat), 50 to 60 percent carbohydrates (mostly complex carbohydrates), and about 10 to 20 percent protein. These amounts could certainly vary from one individual to another (assuming differences in exercise levels) but are generally considered a good starting point for a healthy diet.

MICRONUTRIENTS

Just like macronutrients, vitamins and minerals are essential to life, so they are also considered nutrients. They are needed in such small amounts compared with macronutrients, however, that they are called *micronutrients*.

Because vitamins and minerals are so necessary for health, the US Food and Nutrition Board of the National Research Council (NRC) has formulated recommended consumption levels, called the Recommended Daily Allowances (RDAs). But the amounts cited in these recommendations usually are adequate for maintaining a minimal level of health—that is, basic levels to ward off disease—rather than optimal health. Therefore, any adult not suffering from a specific disorder should be able to obtain more than enough of the RDAs of vitamins and minerals from food or supplement sources. People who are active, under great stress, on restricted diets, mentally or physically ill, taking medication, or recovering from surgery, or those who smoke or consume alcoholic beverages, all need higher than the normal recommended amounts. Women who take oral contraceptives also need increased amounts.

Vitamins and Related Compounds

Vitamins are essential to life. They contribute to good health by regulating metabolism and assisting in biochemical processes that release energy from digested food. Some vitamins are water-soluble vitamins, while some vitamins are fat-soluble vitamins. Water-soluble vitamins must be taken into the body daily, as they cannot be stored and are excreted within one to four days. These include the B vitamins and vitamin C. Fat-soluble vitamins can be stored for longer periods in the body, in fatty tissues and the liver. These include vitamins A, D, E, and K. The body needs both water-soluble and fat-soluble vitamins for proper functioning.

Vitamin A and Beta-Carotene

Of all the micronutrients that are important to visual functioning, the most well-known example is probably vitamin A. Vitamin A is a fat-soluble vitamin that occurs in nature in a variety of chemical forms. It is found as *retinol* in animal tissues and as *beta-carotene* in plants, with the highest amounts present in fruits such as apricots and cantaloupes, and in vegetables such as carrots, pumpkins, sweet potatoes, spinach, squash, and broccoli. You might have noticed that many of these are orange in color—a giveaway that they contain beta-carotene. While retinol is readily absorbed in its natural state by the body, beta-carotene must be broken down before it can function as a vitamin.

Beta-carotene is a *carotenoid* (ka-ROT-en-oyd), which is a class of compounds related to vitamin A. Some carotenoids, such as beta-carotene, can act as precursors of vitamin A. When a food or supplement containing beta-carotene is consumed, the beta-carotene is converted into vitamin A by the liver. According to recent reports, moderate amounts of beta-carotene appears to aid in cancer prevention by scavenging, or neutralizing, *free radicals*, which are molecules that easily react with other molecules and can lead to oxidative damage in the body. (See the inset "Free Radicals and Antioxidants" on page 117.)

Vitamin A is the molecule in the retina that is responsible for the transformation of light energy into nerve impulses. It is therefore critical in the functioning of the eye. A lack of vitamin A can cause some forms of night blindness. Vitamin A enhances immunity, may heal gastrointestinal ulcers, protects against pollution and cancer formation, and assists in the maintenance and repair of mucous tissue. (Since vitamin A is necessary for the maintenance of the mucous lining of various tissues, including the eye, it is also vital to the maintenance of a proper tear level and the prevention of dry eye disease.) It is important in the formation of bones and teeth, aids in fat storage, and protects against colds, influenza, and infections of the kidneys, bladder, lungs, and mucous membranes. Vitamin A also acts as an *antioxidant*, which refers to a substance that can neutralize free radicals.

The upper intestinal tract is the primary area of absorption of vitamin A, since it's here that fat-splitting enzymes and bile salts convert carotene into a usable nutrient. This conversion is stimulated by *thyroxine,* a *thyroid hormone,* which is made by the *thyroid gland.* Once converted into vitamin A, carotene is absorbed the same way as preformed vitamin A. The conversion of carotene into vitamin A is never complete. Approximately one-third of the carotene in food is converted into vitamin A. Less than one-fourth of the carotene in carrots and root vegetables undergoes conversion, and about half of the carotene in leafy green vegetables does. Some unchanged carotene is absorbed into the circulatory system and stored in fat tissues rather than in the liver. Unabsorbed carotene is excreted.

The degree to which carotene is utilized by the body varies with the food source and the way the food is prepared. Cooking, puréeing, and mashing of a vegetable rupture the cell membranes and therefore make the carotene more available for absorption. Factors interfering with the absorption of vitamin A and carotene include strenuous physical activity performed within four hours of consumption of the nutrient, intake of mineral oil, excessive consumption of alcohol, excessive consumption of iron, and the use of cortisone and other medications. The intake of polyunsaturated fatty acids with carotene results in rapid destruction of the carotene unless antioxidants also are present. Even cold weather can hinder the transport and metabolism of vitamin A and carotene.

Approximately 90 percent of the body's vitamin A is stored in the liver, with small amounts deposited in the fat tissues, lungs, kidneys, and retinas of the eyes. Under stressful conditions, the body uses this reserve supply if it doesn't receive enough vitamin A from the diet. Gastrointestinal and liver disorders, infections of any kind, or any condition in which the bile duct is obstructed can limit the body's capacity to retain and use vitamin A. Factors affecting the absorption of vitamin A include the amount of the nutrient consumed, the influence of other substances present in the intestines, and the amount of the vitamin stored in the body. For these reasons, recommended dietary amounts vary for each individual.

A deficiency of vitamin A may be apparent if night blindness, dry hair or skin, dry eyes, or poor growth is present. Other possible results of a vitamin-A deficiency are abscesses in the ears, insomnia, fatigue, reproductive difficulties, sinusitis, pneumonia, frequent colds or other respiratory infections, skin disorders (including acne), and weight loss.

The issue of vitamin A is a controversial topic in the eyecare industry. Taking large amounts of vitamin A over long periods of time can be toxic to the body, mainly the liver. The RDAs for vitamin A are 1,500 international units (IU) for infants and children up to four years old; 3,000 IU for children from four to twelve years old; and 5,000 IU for children over twelve years old and adults. These amounts increase during disease, trauma, pregnancy, and lactation. The requirements vary for people who smoke, who live in highly polluted areas, who easily absorb vitamin A, and who have pneumonia or nephritis (inflammation of the kidney). Increased intakes of vitamins C and E will help to prevent excessive oxidation (free-radical damage) of stored vitamin A.

Research indicates that no more than 50,000 IU per day of vitamin A can be utilized by the body except in therapeutic cases, where up to

100,000 IU is recommended. It has been suggested that the best level is somewhere between 25,000 and 50,000 IU per day. Nevertheless, do not take an excess of vitamin A without first consulting your physician or healthcare practitioner. Toxic levels of vitamin A are associated with abdominal pain, amenorrhea (halt of menstruation), enlargement of the liver or spleen, gastrointestinal disturbances, hair loss, itchiness, joint pain, nausea and vomiting, water on the brain, and small cracks and scales on the lips.

Vitamin C can help prevent the harmful effects of vitamin A toxicity. Overdose is unlikely with beta-carotene, although if you take too much, your skin may turn slightly yellow-orange in color. Excessive beta-carotene, however, has been linked to reduced levels of lutein and zeaxanthin levels in the retina. It seems that these three carotenoids compete for transport around the body. Beta-carotene (being the largest of the molecules) takes precedence and will not allow the lutein and zeaxanthin molecules to get to the retina, where they would protect the retina from high energy blue light. Thus, it is important to make sure that the vitamin A in your supplement is "fully formed" and not "100 percent as beta-carotene." In addition, it is important to take only natural beta-carotene or a natural carotenoid complex.

Supplemental beta-carotene was shown to increase the risk of lung cancer in smokers in a study conducted in Finland, called the "Alpha-Tocopherol, Beta-Carotene Cancer Prevention (ATBC) Study." A second study, "Carotenoid and Retinol Efficacy Trial (CARET)," also found a higher incidence of lung cancer in those people who took a whopping 30 mg of synthetic beta-carotene along with 25,000 IU of pre-formed Vitamin A retinol.

The amounts of supplemental Vitamin A and beta-carotene included in both the ATBC and CARET studies were far beyond the safe upper limits (UL) for daily consumption established by the Food and Nutrition Board at the Institute of Medicine. The UL established by the Institute of Medicine for the combination of pre-formed Vitamin A as retinol, and pro-formed Vitamin A as retinol activity carotenoids (primarily beta-carotene) is 10,000 IU, or approximately 3,000 retinol equivalents (RAE) per day.

At about the same time, the twelve-year-long "Physicians' Health Study (PHS)," involving more than 22,000 physician volunteers, showed no statistical increase in lung cancer rates in doctors who were taking a full-spectrum multivitamin and 50 mg of synthetic beta carotene, even in the 11 percent of physician volunteers who were heavy smokers.

Data in the *American Journal of Epidemiology* clearly suggests that, in fact, smokers who consume small amounts of natural supplemental beta-carotene in combination with a wide variety of supplemental antioxidants actually lower their overall risk of developing lung cancer by 16 percent. Beta-carotene is not vitamin A. It is a rate-limiting pro-formed vitamin A hydrocarbon carotenoid. The body's need for vitamin A is so critical it will convert plant-based hydrocarbon beta-carotene to vitamin A retinol if retinol liver stores are deficient. If there is no retinol deficiency, beta-carotene functions as a powerhouse antioxidant, particularly against retina-damaging singlet oxygen, and does not convert to retinol. Both beta-carotene conversion and retinol conversion also become less efficient with the aging process, so research-focused nutritional biochemists stopped recommending beta-carotene as a sole source of supplemental vitamin A for older men and women years ago.

Vitamin A has been successfully used in the treatment of several eye disorders, including Bitot's spots (white, elevated, sharply outlined patches on the sclera), blurred vision, night blindness, and cataracts. Therapeutic dosages of vitamin A may also be considered in the treatment of glaucoma, dry eye disease, and pink eye.

The Vitamin B Complex

All B vitamins are water-soluble substances that can be cultivated from bacteria, yeast, fungi, or mold. The substances often included in a B-complex supplement are vitamins B_1 (thiamine), B_2 (riboflavin), B_3 (niacin), B_5 (pantothenic acid), B_6 (pyridoxine), B_7 (biotin), B_9 (folic acid), and B_{12} (cyanocobalamin), as well as choline, inositol, and para-aminobenzoic acid (PABA), which are related substances but not actually B vitamins. The grouping of these water-soluble compounds under the term "B complex" is based upon their common sources, their close relationship in vegetable and animal tissues, and their functional relationships.

B-complex vitamins are active in providing the body with energy by converting carbohydrates into glucose, which the body burns to produce energy. They are vital in the metabolism of fat and protein. In addition, the B vitamins are necessary for the normal functioning of the nervous system, and may be the single most important factor in the health of the nerves. They are essential for the maintenance of muscle tone in the gastrointestinal tract, and for the health of the skin, hair, liver, mouth, and eyes.

All of the B vitamins are natural constituents of brewer's yeast, liver, and whole-grain cereals. Brewer's yeast is the richest natural source of the B-complex group. Another important source of B vitamins is intestinal bacteria. These bacteria grow best on milk sugar and small amounts of fat in the diet.

Because of the water solubility of B vitamins, any excess B vitamin is excreted rather than stored. Therefore, B vitamins must be continually replaced. All of the B vitamins, when mixed with saliva, are readily absorbed. Sulfa drugs, barbiturates (sleeping pills), insecticides, and estrogen can create a condition in the digestive tract that can destroy B vitamins. Certain B vitamins are lost through perspiration.

The most important thing to remember is that all B vitamins should be taken together. They are so interrelated in function that a large dose of any one of them may be therapeutically valueless, or it may cause a deficiency of other B vitamins. For example, if you take extra B6, you must take a complete B complex along with it. In nature, we find B vitamins in green vegetables, but nowhere do we find a single B vitamin isolated from the rest. The need for B-complex vitamins increases during infection and stress. Alcoholics and individuals who consume excessive amounts of carbohydrates require higher intakes of the B vitamins for proper metabolism. Coffee uses up the B vitamins. Children and pregnant women need extra B vitamins for normal growth.

B vitamins are so meagerly supplied in the American diet that almost every person in this country lacks some of them. If you are tired, irritable, nervous, depressed, or even suicidal, suspect a vitamin-B deficiency. Gray hair, baldness, acne and other skin problems, poor appetite, insomnia, neuritis (disease of the peripheral nerves), anemia, constipation, and a high cholesterol level also are indicators of a vitamin-B deficiency. One reason there is such a great vitamin-B deficiency in the American population is that we eat so much processed food from which B vitamins have been removed. Another reason for this widespread deficiency is the high amount of sugar we consume, as B vitamins are destroyed by sugar and alcohol.

The B vitamins have been used in the treatment of barbiturate overdose, alcoholic psychosis, and drug-induced delirium. An adequate dose has been found to control migraine headaches and attacks of Meniere's syndrome (a disease of the inner ear). Some heart abnormalities have responded to the use of B-complex vitamins because the nerves affecting the heart need B-complex vitamins for smooth, quiet functioning. Massive dosages of B-complex vitamins have been used to treat polio, improve the condition of hypersensitive children who fail to respond favorably to medications such as Ritalin, and relieve cases of shingles. Nervous individuals and persons working under great amounts of tension or stress can greatly benefit from taking larger than normal doses of the B vitamins.

B vitamins may also help to treat beriberi (caused by a vitamin-B_1 deficiency), pellagra (caused by a deficiency of vitamin B_3), eyelid twitching, double vision, fatigue, skin disorders, cracks at the corners of the mouth, anemia, and dry eye. The following substances are components of the B complex that are most important to eye health.

Vitamin B_1 (Thiamine). Vitamin B_1, also known as thiamine, is a water-soluble vitamin that combines with pyruvic acid to form a coenzyme necessary for the breakdown of carbohydrates into glucose, which is oxidized by the body to produce energy. Thiamine is vulnerable to heat, air, and water in cooking. It is a component of the germ and bran of wheat, the husk of rice, and that portion of all grains which is commercially milled away to give the grain a lighter color and finer texture.

Thiamine enhances circulation, assists in the formation of blood, and aids in the production of hydrochloric acid, which is important for proper digestion. Thiamine also optimizes cognitive activity and brain functioning. It has a positive effect on energy, growth, appetite, and learning capacity, and is needed for muscle tone in the intestines, stomach, and heart. It also acts as an antioxidant, protecting the body from the degenerative effects of aging, alcohol consumption, and smoking.

Thiamine deficiency can lead to inflammation of the optic nerve, called *optic neuritis,* as well as to impairment of the central nervous system. The first signs of thiamine deficiency include fatigue, loss of appetite, irritability, and emotional instability. If the deficiency is not addressed, confusion and loss of memory appear, followed closely by gastric distress, abdominal pain, and constipation.

The RDA for thiamine is 1.1 to 1.4 milligrams a day. A thiamine intake of 1.4 milligrams daily is recommended during pregnancy and lactation. The need for thiamine increases during severe diarrhea, fever, stress, and surgery. Thiamine has no known toxic side effects.

The richest food sources of thiamine include brown rice, egg yolks, fish, legumes, liver, pork, poultry, rice bran, wheat germ, and whole grains. Other sources include asparagus, brewer's yeast, broccoli, Brussels sprouts, dulse, kelp, most nuts, oatmeal, plums, dried prunes, raisins, spirulina, and watercress. Herbs that contain thiamine include alfalfa, bladderwrack, burdock, catnip, cayenne, chamomile, chickweed, eyebright, fennel, fenugreek, hops, nettle, oat straw, parsley, peppermint, raspberry, red clover, rose hips, sage, yarrow, and yellow dock.

Vitamin B2 (Riboflavin). Vitamin B_2, also known as riboflavin, is a water-soluble vitamin that occurs naturally in the same foods containing other B vitamins. Riboflavin is stable to heat, oxidation, and acid, but disintegrates in the presence of alkalis or light, especially ultraviolet (UV) light.

Riboflavin functions as part of a group of enzymes involved in the breakdown and utilization of carbohydrates, fat, and protein. It is necessary for cell respiration because it works with enzymes in the utilization of cell oxygen. Riboflavin supports mitochondrial energy production by stimulating metabolism of fat, carbohydrates, and protein. (The mitochondria are parts of the cell known as the "powerhouses" of the cell, as they are essential to energy production in the cell.) It is required for red blood cell formation and respiration, antibody production, growth, and reproduction. It also helps in the prevention of many types of eye disorders, including bloodshot eyes, itchy or burning eyes, cataracts, and abnormal sensitivity to light. It is also necessary for the maintenance of good vision, skin, nails, and hair. Undernourished women at the end of pregnancy often suffer from conditions such as visual disturbances, burning eyes, and excessive tearing.

Riboflavin deficiency is the most common vitamin deficiency in the United States. This deficiency can result from long-established faulty dietary habits, food idiosyncrasies, alcoholism, arbitrarily selected diets used for the relief of digestive problems, or prolonged dietary restriction. The most common symptoms of a lack of B_2 are cracks and sores in the corners of the mouth; a red, sore tongue; a feeling of grit or sand on the insides of the eyelids; burning eyes; eye fatigue; dilated pupils; corneal changes; light sensitivity; lesions on the lips; scaling around the nose, mouth, or forehead; trembling; sluggishness; dizziness; and vaginal itchiness.

The RDA for riboflavin is 1.6 milligrams for adult males and 1.2 milligrams for adult females. During pregnancy and lactation, the requirement goes up to 1.5 milligrams and 1.7 milligrams, respectively. There are no known toxic side effects associated with the use of riboflavin. Excessive amounts of B_2, however, make the retina extremely sensitive to light, and prolonged ingestion of large doses of any one of the B-complex vitamins, including riboflavin, may result in high urinary losses of other B vitamins. Therefore, it is important to take a complete B complex along with any single B vitamin.

Vitamin B₃ (Niacin). Niacin is another member of the B-complex family of vitamins, and is also a water-soluble vitamin. It is more stable than either thiamine or riboflavin, and is remarkably resistant to heat, light, air, acids, and alkalis. As a coenzyme, niacin assists enzymes in the breakdown and utilization of protein, fat, and carbohydrates. Niacin is effective at improving circulation and reducing blood-cholesterol levels. It is vital to the proper functioning of the nervous system, and for the formation and maintenance of healthy tongue, digestive system tissues, and skin.

Relatively small amounts of pure niacin are present in most foods. The niacin equivalent listed in dietary tables refers either to pure niacin or to tryptophan, an amino acid that can be converted into niacin by the body. Lean meats, poultry, fish, and peanuts are rich sources of both niacin and tryptophan, as are such dietary supplements as brewer's yeast, wheat germ, and desiccated liver. Niacin is difficult to obtain except from these foods.

The RDAs suggest that the daily allowance of niacin be based on caloric intake, with 6.6 milligrams of niacin recommended for every 1,000 calories. There have been no toxic side effects reported for niacin, but taking extremely large doses can cause tingling and itchy sensations, intense flushing of the skin, and throbbing in the head. There is also a possibility of a condition called *cystoid maculopathy*, in which the macula of the retina swells, causing visual distortions. This condition is reversible when the overdose is stopped.

Excessive consumption of sugar and starches depletes the body's supply of niacin, as does taking certain antibiotics. The symptoms of niacin deficiency are many. In the early stages, they include muscular weakness, general fatigue, appetite loss, indigestion, and various skin eruptions. Niacin deficiency may also cause bad breath, small ulcers, canker sores, insomnia, irritability, nausea, vomiting, recurring headaches, tender gums, strain, tension, or deep depression.

Vitamin B₅ (Pantothenic Acid). Pantothenic acid, also known as vitamin B_5 is required for the conversion of carbohydrates, fat, and protein into usable energy for the body. It is necessary for the synthesis of red blood cells and steroid metabolism, and plays a vital role in the synthesis of fatty acids, cholesterol, and other biological compounds. It is the precursor of coenzyme A (CoA), which is necessary for mitochondrial energy production.

Pantothenic-acid deficiency results in diminished adrenal gland functioning. A variety of metabolic problems will also manifest themselves. Fatigue is common along with depression and problems associated with the digestive system. There will also be loss of nerve functioning and problems with blood sugar metabolism, with hypoglycemia, or low blood sugar, being the most common. Pantothenic-acid deficiency can reduce immune system responses, increasing the risk of infection. Other symptoms include skin problems, insomnia, coordination problems, muscle cramps, and worsening of allergy symptoms.

Vitamin B₆ (Pyridoxine). Vitamin B_6 is a water-soluble vitamin consisting of three related compounds: pyridoxine, pyrdoxinal, and pyridoxamine. It is required for the proper absorption of vitamin B_{12}, and for the production of hydrochloric acid and magnesium. Pyridoxine plays an important role as a coenzyme in the breakdown and utilization of carbohydrates, fat, and protein. It is required for the production of antibodies and red blood cells. In addition, it facilitates the release of glycogen for energy from the liver and muscles. Vitamin B_6 is converted to pryidoxal-5 phosphate, which is directly involved in mitochondrial biosynthesis.

Vitamin B_6 helps to maintain the balance between sodium and potassium, which regulate bodily fluids and promote the normal functioning of the nervous and musculoskeletal systems. The best sources of vitamin B_6 are meats and whole grains, specifically desiccated liver and brewer's yeast.

According to the RDAs, the daily allowance of vitamin B_6 is based on protein intake. Adults need 2 milligrams of pyridoxine for every 100 grams of protein they consume per day. Children need 0.6 to 1.2 milligrams for every 100 grams of protein they consume. The need for vitamin B_6 doubles during pregnancy, lactation, exposure to radiation, cardiac failure, aging, and use of oral contraceptives.

Approximately 10 percent of the US population consumes less than half of the B_6 RDA. Recent epidemiological studies have indicated an association between B_6 deficiency and increased cancer. In cases of vitamin-B_6 deficiency, there is low blood sugar and low glucose tolerance, resulting in sensitivity to insulin. Deficiency may also cause loss of hair, water retention during pregnancy, cracks around the mouth and eyes, numbness and cramps in the arms and legs, slow learning, visual disturbances, neuritis, arthritis, heart disorders, and increased urination.

Vitamin B_{12} (Cyanocobalamin). B complex member vitamin B_{12} is unique in that it is the first cobalt-containing substance found to be essential for longevity. In addition, it is the only vitamin that contains essential mineral elements. Vitamin B_{12} cannot be made synthetically but rather must be grown, like penicillin, in bacteria or molds. One of the only foods in which B_{12} occurs naturally in substantial amounts is animal protein. Therefore, vegetarians and vegans are frequently low in vitamin B_{12}. At the same time, high blood levels of folic acid, also common in vegetarians, can mask a vitamin-B_{12} deficiency. Liver is the best source of B_{12}, and kidney, muscle meats, fish, and dairy products are other good sources.

Vitamin B_{12} is necessary for the normal metabolism of nerve tissue, and is involved in protein, fat, and carbohydrate metabolism. Vitamin B_{12} is taken into the mitochondria and plays an important role in amino acid metabolism. The actions of B_{12} are closely related to those of four amino acids, vitamin B_5, and vitamin C. Vitamin B_{12} also helps iron to function better in the body, and aids folic acid in the synthesis of choline.

The human requirement for vitamin B_{12} is minute, but the vitamin is still essential to health. The RDA for vitamin B_{12} is 3 micrograms for adults, and 4 micrograms for pregnant and lactating women. Infants require a daily intake of approximately 3 micrograms, and growing children need about 1 to 2 micrograms. No cases of vitamin-B_{12} toxicity have ever been reported.

A B_{12} deficiency has been shown to affect 10 to 15 percent of individuals over the age of sixty in the United States. Patients with B_{12} deficiency exhibit megaloblastic anemia and often hyperhomocysteinemia, which has been associated with an increased risk of *macular degeneration*. The symptoms of a vitamin-B_{12} deficiency may take five or six years to appear. Deficiency of the vitamin is usually due to a lack of the intrinsic factor, a glycoprotein necessary for the absorption of B_{12}. Deficiency begins with changes in the nervous system such as soreness and weakness in the legs and arms, diminished reflex response and sensory perception, difficulty walking and speaking, and jerking of the limbs. The condition known as *tobacco amblyopia,* a loss of vision due to tobacco poisoning, has been improved with injections of vitamin B_{12}, whether or not the patient stopped smoking. The symptoms of tobacco amblyopia include blackouts, headaches, and loss of focusing ability.

Choline. Although not technically a B vitamin, choline is included in the B-complex. It functions with inositol, also considered a B-complex vitamin, as a basic constituent of lecithin, an essential type of fat. It is present in the bodies of all living cells, and is widely distributed in animal and plant tissues. Lecithin is the richest source of choline, but other rich dietary sources are egg yolks, liver, brewer's yeast, and wheat germ.

Choline appears to be associated primarily with the utilization of fat and cholesterol in the body. It prevents fat from accumulating in the liver, and facilitates its movement into the cells. It is essential for the health of the liver and kidneys.

Choline is also essential for the health of the myelin sheaths of the nerves. The myelin sheaths are the principal components of the nerve fibers, and are the primary target of multiple sclerosis, in which the sheaths of the nerves degenerate. Choline plays an important role in the transmission of the nerve impulses. The eye is one of the most highly innervated organs in the body, so adequate levels of choline are critical for proper eye functioning.

The daily requirements for choline unknown. The average American adult diet contains about 500 to 900 milligrams of choline a day.

Vitamin C

Vitamin C, also known as ascorbic acid, is a water-soluble nutrient. Although fairly stable in acid solutions, it is normally the least stable of the vitamins, and is very sensitive to oxygen. Its potency can be lost through exposure to light, heat, or air, all of which stimulate the activity of the oxidative enzymes.

The primary function of vitamin C is to maintain the body's collagen, a protein necessary for the formation of the connective tissue in the skin, ligaments, bones, and, most importantly for our purposes, sclera of the eye. Vitamin C plays a role in the healing of wounds and burns because it facilitates the formation of connective tissue in scars. Vitamin C also aids in the formation of red blood cells and the prevention of hemorrhaging. In addition, vitamin C fights bacterial infection and reduces the effects on the body of some allergens. For these reasons, vitamin C is frequently used in the prevention and treatment of the common cold.

Vitamin C is present in most fresh fruit and vegetables. Natural vitamin C dietary supplements are prepared from rose hips, acerola cherries, green peppers, and citrus fruit.

The level of ascorbic acid in the blood reaches a maximum about two or three hours after the ingestion of a moderate quantity of the nutrient and then decreases as the vitamin is eliminated in the urine and through perspiration. Most vitamin C is out of the body in three to four hours. Because vitamin C is a "stress vitamin," it is used up even more rapidly under stressful conditions. Humans, apes, and guinea pigs are the only animals that must obtain vitamin C from their food because they are unable to meet the body's needs by synthesis alone. Ascorbic acid is readily absorbed from the gastrointestinal tract into the bloodstream. Two factors that influence its absorption are the manner in which the vitamin is administered and the presence of other substances in the intestinal tract. The normal human body, when fully saturated, contains about 5,000 milligrams of vitamin C, of which 30 milligrams are found in the adrenal glands, 200 milligrams in extracellular fluids, and the rest in various concentrations throughout the cells of the entire body.

Vitamin C promotes bone and tooth formation while protecting the dentine and pulp of teeth. Some types of viral and bacterial infections are prevented or cured by vitamin C. One school of thought regarding the effects of vitamin C on the development of nearsightedness is that the vitamin fortifies the sclera of the eye, being connective tissue. If there is a lack of vitamin C for an extended period, especially during the high growth years, the eye structure will weaken, allowing the pressure inside the eye to expand the length of the eye, which leads to nearsightedness. In addition, it is a fact that the fluid filling the anterior chamber of the eye—between the cornea and the lens—maintains a vitamin-C level approximately twenty times higher than that of the blood plasma. This is considered significant in the nutrition of the lens, which has no blood supply and depends on the aqueous fluid for its nourishment. It only stands to reason that the level of vitamin C should be upheld or increased as we age to maintain a clear and healthy lens within the eye.

The RDA for vitamin C is 45 milligrams for adults. The now-famous Dr. Linus Pauling, however, suggested that the optimal daily intake of vitamin C for most human adults is from 2,300 to 9,000 milligrams. This wide range takes into account differences in weight, activity level, metabolism, ailments, and age.

Toxicity symptoms usually do not occur with high intakes of vitamin C because the body simply discharges whatever it cannot use. Nevertheless, a daily intake of 5,000 to 15,000 milligrams may cause side effects in some people. The toxicity symptoms of vitamin C include a slight burning sensation during urination, loose bowels, and skin rashes.

The body's ability to absorb vitamin C is reduced by smoking, stress, high fever, prolonged intake of antibiotics or cortisone, inhalation of petroleum fumes, and ingestion of aspirin or other painkillers. Baking soda destroys vitamin C, as does cooking with copper utensils. The signs of deficiency include shortness of breath, impaired digestion, poor lactation, bleeding gums, weakened tooth enamel or dentine, tendency to bruising, swollen or painful joints, nosebleeds, anemia, lowered resistance to infections, and slow healing of wounds. Severe deficiency results in scurvy.

Vitamin D

Vitamin D is a fat-soluble vitamin that can be acquired both from food and through exposure to sunlight. It is known as the "sunshine vitamin" because the sun's UV rays activate a form of cholesterol present in the skin, converting the substance to vitamin D.

Vitamin D aids in the absorption of calcium from the intestinal tract, and in the breakdown and assimilation of phosphorus, which is required for bone formation. In the mucous membranes, it helps to synthesize enzymes that are involved in the active transport of available calcium.

Vitamin D is necessary for normal growth in children, for without it, the bones and teeth do not calcify properly.

Adults also benefit from vitamin D. It is valuable for maintaining a stable nervous system, normal heart action, and normal blood clotting, as all these functions are related to the body's supply and utilization of calcium and phosphorus. Vitamin D is best utilized by the body when taken with vitamin A. Fish-liver oils are the best natural sources of vitamins A and D.

Most of the body's need for vitamin D can be met by sufficient exposure to sunlight and ingestion of small amounts of food. The sun's action on the skin can be inhibited, however, by such factors as air pollution, clouds, window glass, clothing, and, of course, sunscreen. The RDA for vitamin D is set at 400 IU per day, which should meet the requirements of most healthy individuals who are not regularly exposed to UV light.

Being a fat-soluble vitamin means that vitamin D can be stored in the body. Excessive blood levels of this vitamin can cause a rise in the blood levels of calcium and phosphorus, and excessive excretion of calcium in the urine. This leads to calcification of the soft tissues and of the walls of the blood vessels and kidney tubules, a condition known as hypercalcemia. The symptoms of acute overdose include increased frequency of urination, loss of appetite, nausea, vomiting, diarrhea, muscular weakness, dizziness, weariness, and calcification of the soft tissues of the heart, blood vessels, and lungs. These symptoms disappear within a few days of lowering the dosage of vitamin D or discontinuing its use completely.

A deficiency of vitamin D leads to inadequate absorption of calcium from the intestinal tract and retention of phosphorus in the kidneys. The inability of the soft bones to withstand the stress of the body's weight results in skeletal malformations. Rickets, a bone disorder in children, is a direct result of vitamin-D deficiency. Adult rickets, called osteomalacia, can also occur. One study showed that vitamin-D deficiency might lead to nearsightedness. An imbalance of this vitamin with calcium is at the root of this disorder. Other possible effects are *keratoconus* (cone-shaped cornea), pink eye, cataracts, and arteriosclerosis.

Vitamin E

Vitamin E, a fat-soluble vitamin, is composed of two groups of compounds called tocopherols and tocotrienols. Eight forms exist: four of tocopherol—alpha, beta, delta, and gamma—and four of tocotrienol: alpha, beta, delta, and gamma. Of these, alpha tocopherol is the most popular and has the greatest nutritional and biological values. The tocopherols occur in the highest concentrations in cold-pressed vegetable oils, whole raw seeds and nuts, and soybeans. Wheat germ oil is the source from which vitamin E was first obtained. The tocotrienols have fewer effects but might lower cholesterol and provide some heart health benefits.

Vitamin E is an antioxidant, which means it opposes the oxidation of substances in the body. It plays an essential role in the cellular respiration of muscles, especially the cardiac and skeletal muscles. It makes it possible for these muscles and their nerves to function with less oxygen, thereby increasing their endurance and stamina. It also causes dilation of blood vessels, permitting a fuller flow of blood to the heart, as well as to the other organs. Vitamin E also helps to counter the gradual decline in metabolic processes during aging. As a diuretic, vitamin E helps to lower elevated blood pressure. It protects against the damaging effects of many environmental poisons in the air, water, and food.

Vitamin E is effective against the formation of elevated scar tissue on the surface of the body and within the body. In ointment form, vitamin E can aid in the healing of burned tissue, skin ulcers, and abrasions. It also lessens the formation of scars. It is also helpful in counteracting premature aging of the skin. It is useful to apply vitamin E to the skin in ointment form while also taking it orally, because it affects cell formation by replacing the cells on the outer layer of the skin.

Several substances interfere with, or even cause a depletion of, vitamin E in the body. For example, when iron (especially the inorganic form) and vitamin E are administered together, the absorption of both is impaired. Chlorine in drinking water, ferric chloride, rancid oil or fat, and inorganic iron compounds destroy vitamin E in the body. Mineral oil used as a laxative depletes vitamin E. Large amounts of polyunsaturated fats or oils in the diet increase the oxidation rate of vitamin E. The more unsaturated fats or oils that are consumed, the more vitamin E is necessary.

Vitamin E has many beneficial effects. It works to treat and prevent heart diseases, such as coronary thrombosis, a heart attack caused by vessels being blocked by blood clots. Vitamin E causes arterial blood clots to disintegrate. Angina, a condition in which chest pain results from an insufficient supply of blood to the heart tissues, is successfully treated with alpha tocopherol. Vitamin E is beneficial to persons with atherosclerosis, which refers to a buildup of plaque along the walls of arteries, if used as a therapy before irreparable damage occurs. It relieves pain in the extremities, speeds up blood flow, and reduces clotting tendencies.

Vitamin E therapy has been suggested as beneficial in a number of other conditions, including bursitis (inflammation of a bursa resulting in joint pain), gout (defective uric-acid metabolism), arthritis, nearsightedness, strabismus, varicose veins, thrombosis (thickening of the blood resulting in blood clots), phlebitis (inflammation of the wall of a vein), nephritis, and even headaches.

The RDA for vitamin E is based upon metabolic body size and level of polyunsaturated fatty acids in the diet, rather than upon weight or caloric intake. The requirements increase along with any increases in the amount of polyunsaturated fatty acids consumed. The RDA is 4 to 5 IU daily for infants, 7 to 12 IU for children and adolescents, 15 IU for adult males, 12 IU for adult females, and 15 IU for pregnant or lactating females. Many nutritionists, however, consider these allowances exceedingly low.

The first sign of a vitamin-E deficiency is the rupture of red blood cells, resulting from the cells' increased fragility. A deficiency could result in a reduction of membrane stability and shrinkage of collagen. In addition, a tendency toward muscular wasting or abnormal fat deposits in the muscles, or an increased demand for oxygen may occur in a state of vitamin-E deficiency. Essential fatty acids are also altered so that blood cells break down and hemoglobin formation is impaired. The body's ability to utilize several amino acids may also be impaired, and the level of functioning of the pituitary and adrenal glands may be reduced. Iron absorption and hemoglobin formation may also be impaired.

Severe deficiency can cause damage to the kidneys and liver. A prolonged deficiency of vitamin E can cause faulty absorption of fat and the fat-soluble vitamins. Poor utilization of vitamin E or an increased demand for it can cause anemia.

There has been a concern in one research study about vitamin-E overdosing as a supplement to the diet. This isolated finding applied only to an older group of patients (over the age of seventy) with a long history of heart disease, stroke, or diabetes, and who were also taking a combination of medications, including ACE inhibitors, calcium channel blockers, anti-platelet agents, and lipid-lowering agents during the course of the study. A significant percentage of study participants were also cigarette smokers, further clouding the issue.

The Council for Responsible Nutrition continues to support the safe upper limits of vitamin E established by the Food and Nutrition Board at the Institute of Medicine. The published safe daily upper limits are 1,000 IU of synthetic Vitamin E and 1,500 IU of natural vitamin E, however, under normal circumstances a daily supplement of 200 IU is adequate.

Free Radicals and Antioxidants

Oxygen splits into single atoms with unpaired electrons in the body. Electrons like to be in pairs, so these atoms are called free radicals. These molecules circulate throughout the body, seeking out other electrons so they can become paired up once again. This act of pairing, however, pulls an electron from another molecule, creating yet another free radical. This process then repeats, causing damage to cells, proteins, and DNA, leading to a condition known as oxidative stress.

Free radicals are associated with many diseases, including cancer, atherosclerosis, Alzheimer's disease, Parkinson's disease, and many others. They have also been shown to advance the process of aging.

Free radicals are the natural byproducts of chemical processes such as metabolism. They may be considered waste products from various chemical reactions in the cell that can harm the cells in the body if allowed to accumulate. Substances that generate free radicals can also be found in the food we eat, medicines we take, air pollution, and even in the water we drink. These substances include fried foods, alcohol, tobacco smoke, pesticides, and air pollutants.

Antioxidants keep free radicals balanced. Antioxidants are molecules in cells that prevent free radicals from taking electrons and causing damage. They are able to give an electron to a free radical without becoming destabilized, thus stopping the free-radical chain reaction. Antioxidants clean up free-radical waste in cells. Some of the more popular antioxidants include beta-carotene, lutein, resveratrol, vitamin C, vitamin E, and lycopene.

Researchers also estimated that over 80 percent of the American public does not get even the minimal required amount of vitamin E from their diet. One distinguished vitamin-E researcher commented, "Vitamin E deficiency could make us more prone to atherosclerosis or diseases that involve an enhanced production of oxygen radicals. Renegade radical molecules can rampage throughout cells, destroying lipids, proteins, and DNA. By disarming oxygen radicals, vitamin E may act as an insurance policy against oxidative stress."

Acetyl-L-Carnitine (ALC)

Acetyl-L-carnitine is a delivery form of the amino acid L-carnitine. It transports omega-3 long-chain fatty acids across the mitochondrial membranes into the mitochondria and transports small-chain and medium-chain fatty acids out of the mitochondria in order to maintain normal coenzyme A levels in these specialized structures within the cell. This is particularly important for maintenance of retinal health.

Acetyl-L-carnitine levels may decrease with advancing age. Because it is not an essential nutrient, however, true deficiencies do not occur. Most research involving acetyl-L-carnitine has used 500 milligrams three times per day, though some research has used double this amount.

Side effects from taking acetyl-L-carnitine are uncommon, although skin rash, increased appetite, nausea, vomiting, agitation, and body odor have been reported in people taking this supplement.

Alpha-Lipoic Acid (ALA)

Alpha-lipoic acid is both water- and fat-soluble and is a vital cofactor for production of enzymes necessary for mitochondrial functioning. ALA works together with other antioxidants such as vitamins C and E. It is important for growth, helps to prevent cell damage, and helps the body rid itself of harmful substances.

Several studies suggest that treatment with ALA may help reduce pain, burning, itchiness, tingling, and numbness in people who have nerve damage (called peripheral neuropathy) caused by diabetes. Alpha-lipoic acid has been used for years for this purpose in Europe. Other studies have shown that alpha-lipoic acid speeds the removal of glucose (sugar) from the blood of people with diabetes.

Because alpha-lipoic acid can pass easily into the brain, it has protective effects on brain and nerve tissue and shows promise as a treatment for stroke and other brain disorders involving free-radical damage. Animal studies have shown positive results, but more research is needed to understand whether this benefit applies to people as well.

Additional conditions for which alpha-lipoic acid may prove useful include heart failure, human immunodeficiency virus (HIV), cataracts, and glaucoma. More research is underway in these areas. Good food sources of alpha-lipoic acid include spinach, broccoli, beef, yeast (particularly brewer's yeast), and certain organ meats (such as the kidney and heart).

Astaxanthin

Of all the carotenoids in the diet, astaxanthin is the most powerful natural biological antioxidant. It is closely related to the other carotenoids but is the longest molecule of the group. Because of its length, it is able to span the membrane of the cell, providing support and giving it superior ability to control inflammation. A significant area of effectiveness for astaxanthin is in muscles.

There are many muscles in and around the eyes, so adequate levels of the carotenoid astaxanthin have been shown to help reduce eyestrain. The ciliary muscle, which controls the focusing of the lens benefits from increased levels of astaxanthin. The *extraocular muscles* (muscles outside the eyeball), which control the eye movements, are also beneficiaries of the effect of astaxanthin. One of the main symptoms of eyestrain is "tiring," which usually points to a problem with convergence, where the eyes aim together at a near target. Research has also shown that astaxanthin also increases blood flow into retinal tissue.

The best sources of astaxanthin are the ones where the molecule is from extracted from algae in an indoor setting, where it is protected from pollutants and temperature changes, assuring absolute purity and highest quality. Studies have shown that an intake of just 6 milligrams per day is an effective dose of astaxanthin.

Bioflavonoids

Bioflavonoids, sometimes known as vitamin P, are water-soluble compounds composed of a group of brightly colored substances that often appear in fruits and vegetables as companions to vitamin C. The members of the group are citrin, hesperidin, rutin, the flavones, and the flavonals.

Bioflavonoids were first discovered as substances in the white part, not the juice, of citrus fruits. The edible part of citrus fruits contains ten times more bioflavonoids than the strained juice. Sources of the bioflavonoids include lemons, grapes, plums, black currants, grapefruits, apricots, buckwheat, cherries, blackberries, and rose hips.

Bioflavonoids are essential for the proper absorption and use of vitamin C. They assist vitamin C in keeping collagen in healthy condition. They also have the ability to increase the strength of capillaries and to regulate capillaries' permeability. These actions help to prevent hemorrhages and ruptures in capillaries and connective tissue, and to build a protective barrier against infection. The blood-vessel leakage that occurs within the retina of the eye may be reduced to some degree by the use of a vitamin C-bioflavonoid combination.

The absorption and storage properties, daily requirements, deficiency symptoms, and body utilization of bioflavonoids are all similar to those of vitamin C.

Cannabidiol (CBD)

Cannabidiol, or more commonly known as CBD, is a promising phytocannabinoid. This phytocannabinoid is found in agricultural hemp. It is widely recognized for its benefits to human and animal health, and is capable of affecting nearly every biological process. CBD is non-psychotoxic, in that is it does not result in feelings of euphoria. It also has a remarkable safety profile. Since its discovery in 1992, researchers have been investigating the existence of a central regulatory system called the "endocannabinoid system," or ECS.

The ECS is made up of cannabinoid receptors and is one of the most important physiologic systems involved in establishing and maintaining human health. Endocannabinoids and their receptors are found throughout the body, including the eye. In each tissue, cannabinoids perform different tasks, but the goal is always the same: homeostasis, maintaining a stable internal environment despite fluctuations in the external environment.

Hemp is a form of cannabis that does not contain any significant levels of THC—the molecule that creates the psychoactive "high" that people experience from smoking the other forms of cannabis. Hemp has been wrongly classified as an herb with no medicinal value. The active medicinal molecule is cannabidiol, or CBD.

In the eye, there are receptors on cells that are activated by both THC and CBD molecules. The THC molecule has been shown to lower eye pressure in patients with glaucoma, a disease where the pressure inside the eye rises and leads to death of the optic nerve. CBD molecule receptors are located in the membrane behind the retina, where the process of macular degeneration likely begins. Thus, taking CBD might have an application in this disease. More research is needed to confirm this action, but the science is strong regarding the neuroprotective and antioxidant actions of CBD.

Since CBD is known to ease inflammation, it can be a good supplement for those with eyestrain issues.

Coenzyme Q_{10} (CoQ_{10})

Coenzyme Q_{10}, or CoQ_{10}, is a fat-soluble compound primarily synthesized by the body and also consumed in the diet. It is required for mitochondrial energy synthesis. The primary function of CoQ_{10} is as a catalyst for metabolism—the complex chain of chemical reactions during which food is broken down into packets of energy that the body can use.

Acting in conjunction with enzymes, this compound speeds up the vital metabolic process, providing the energy that the cells need to digest food, heal wounds, maintain healthy muscles, and perform countless other bodily functions. Because of this nutrient's essential role in energy production, it's not surprising that it is found in every cell in the body. It is especially abundant in the energy-intensive cells of the heart. In addition, CoQ_{10} acts as an antioxidant, much like vitamins C and E, helping to neutralize cell-damaging free radicals.

CoQ_{10} may even play a role in preventing cancer, heart attacks, and other diseases linked to free-radical damage. It's also used as a general energy enhancer and anti-aging supplement. Because levels of this compound diminish with age (and with certain diseases), some doctors recommend daily supplementation beginning about age forty. Statin drugs, often prescribed for elevated cholesterol levels, deplete CoQ_{10} levels, therefore CoQ_{10} supplements (about 100 milligrams daily) should be routinely taken with all statin drugs.

Lutein

Lutein (LOO-teen) is similar to beta-carotene and is found in spinach, kale, and other vegetables and fruit. However, unlike beta-carotene, it does not convert to vitamin A, but it does serve as a potent antioxidant. Lutein makes up a large portion of the yellow pigment in the retina, and appears to protect the macula in particular. Research shows that higher dietary levels of lutein (and zeaxanthin) are associated with greater protection of the macula, which can help to prevent macular degeneration. Lutein and zeaxanthin are also found in the crystalline lens, and so may contribute to better protection of the lens and lessen the likelihood of cataract formation.

The body is unable to manufacture lutein. Eating foods containing lutein or consuming dietary supplements that contain lutein is the only way for your body to get it. Within the eye, lutein is highly concentrated in the macular region of the retina and is dispersed in lesser amounts throughout the entire retina, iris, ciliary body, and lens. There is currently no recommended daily intake level for lutein. Research suggests that a minimum of 6 to 10 milligrams a day of lutein from dark green leafy vegetables or other sources is necessary to realize its health benefits. Even if you eat a balanced diet, you would need a large bowl of fresh spinach to get about 6 milligrams of lutein. There are no reports of safety concerns with the intake of large amounts of lutein but also no additional benefits associated larger amounts.

Zeaxanthin

Zeaxanthin (zee-ah-ZAN-thin) is a very close "cousin" of lutein. Its role is to help protect the eye from the harmful high-energy, blue-wave light in the same way sunglasses protect our eyes from sun glare. Zeaxanthin also protects the eye's sensitive macula and helps the eye repair itself. In fact, studies have shown that the portion of the macula with the highest concentration of zeaxanthin is the last to degenerate. The highest density of zeaxanthin is at the very center of the macula, thus affording it the greatest protection. There are also no recommended daily intake levels for zeaxanthin but a recommended amount is 10 milligrams daily for anyone diagnosed with macular degeneration and 4 milligrams for those taking it as a preventative measure.

Another function of zeaxanthin is to reduce glare, since it absorbs the greatly scattered blue light that reaches the retina. This function will also reduce the tendency for eyestrain, as the eye will experience less glare. This effect will lead to a sharper image on the retina and therefore less eyestrain.

Carrots and Eyesight

When discussing nutrition for good eyesight, most people remember being told as children of the beneficial role that carrots play. But do carrots really matter in the maintenance of good vision? Let us look at how this concept was developed.

Carotenoids are a class of mainly yellow, orange, or red fat-soluble pigments, which give color to plant parts. They are "phytochemicals," and are found in the cells of a wide variety of plants, algae, and bacteria. They help plants absorb light energy for use in photosynthesis (converting sunlight to energy). Carotenoids are beneficial antioxidants that can protect you from disease and enhance your immune system. One class of carotenoids, known as provitamin A carotenoids, can be converted into vitamin A, which is essential for growth, immune system functioning, and eye health.

Carrots contain one of the provitamin A carotenoids called beta-carotene (from which the term "carrot" derives). Beta-carotene is a strongly colored orange pigment abundant in plants and fruits, and especially carrots. Beta-carotene may be converted into vitamin A in the body, and vitamin A is important in the proper functioning of the retina. It seems to follow that, since vitamin A is needed by the retina, then increasing beta-carotene intake will lead to better eyesight. But it is not quite that simple!

First, if your liver has adequate vitamin A in storage (which all Americans have), then there is no need to convert more beta-carotene into vitamin A. The body maintains this balance. Second, the process of beta-carotene conversion decreases with age. One issue with excessive beta-carotene is that it competes with other similar molecules for transport around the body. We know that lutein and zeaxanthin (similar molecules) must be transported to the retina. Excess beta-carotene from the diet might impinge the transport of the lutein and zeaxanthin and leave the eye under-protected.

Therefore, the bottom line is that beta-carotene is not an adequate substitute for the preformed retinal palmitate form of vitamin A for eye health. Eating some carrots is still a good idea to stay healthy, though.

Mesozeaxanthin

Another carotenoid is mesozeaxanthin. It is again very similar to the other carotenoids lutein and zeaxanthin but is rarely found in nature as a dietary ingredient. The most common food sources of mesozeaxanthin are fish skin, turtle fat, and shrimp shells, thus it is not readily available in the diet. Mesozeaxanthin is created within the body from the conversion of lutein, so if you have adequate levels of lutein in your system, most likely mesozeaxanthin will be produced and deposited in the central macular area of the retina. Thus, it is likely unnecessary to take a supplement that contains mesozeaxanthin.

Minerals

Minerals are nutrients that exist in the body and in food, in organic and inorganic combinations. Approximately seventeen minerals are essential in human nutrition. Although minerals make up only 4 or 5 percent of a human body's weight, they are vital to overall mental and physical well-being. All of tissues and internal fluids of living things contain various quantities of minerals. Minerals are constituents of the bones, teeth, soft tissue, muscle, blood, and nerve cells. They are important in maintaining the physiological processes, strengthening the skeletal structure, and preserving the vigor of the heart, the brain, and all of the muscle and nerve systems.

Physical and emotional stress can cause a strain on the body's supply of minerals. A mineral deficiency often results in illness, which may be corrected by adding the missing minerals back into the diet.

Calcium

Calcium is the most abundant mineral in the body. About 99 percent of calcium in the body is deposited in bones and teeth, with the remainder found in soft tissues. To function properly, calcium must be accompanied by magnesium, phosphorus, and vitamins A, C, and D. Calcium is stored in mitochondria and participates in cellular calcium signaling. Calcium is also a required cofactor in several mitochondrial proteins, including dehydrogenates (enzymes that take up hydrogen).

Calcium absorption is very inefficient, with usually only 20 to 30 percent of ingested calcium being absorbed. When it needs calcium, however, the body can absorb it more effectively. Therefore, the greater the need for calcium and the smaller the dietary supply, the more efficient the absorption. Absorption is also increased during periods of rapid growth. Calcium absorption depends upon the presence of adequate amounts of vitamin D, which works with the parathyroid hormone to regulate the amount of calcium in the blood. Phosphorus is needed in at least the same amount as calcium. Vitamins A and C are also necessary for calcium absorption. Fat consumed in moderate amounts and moving slowly through the digestive tract facilitates absorption. A high intake of protein also aids in the absorption of calcium.

There is a possibility of "over-calcification" with the ingestion of excessive amounts of calcium over a long period of time. This condition can lead to kidney stones, mitral valve disease, and calcification of the small and large blood vessels (which include those found in eyes).

Iron

Iron is part of hemoglobin, the oxygen-carrying component of blood. Iron-deficient people tire easily because their bodies are starved for oxygen. Iron is also part of myoglobin, which helps muscle cells to store oxygen. Without enough iron, ATP (the fuel the body runs on) cannot be properly synthesized. As a result, some iron-deficient people become fatigued even when their hemoglobin levels are normal.

Although iron is part of the antioxidant enzyme catalase, it is not generally considered an antioxidant because too much iron can cause oxidative damage. An increase in consumption of iron can increase the risk of cardiac disease as well as problems with blood vessels in the eyes. In general, most iron can be accumulated in a good diet and the use of iron supplements is most often not needed.

Magnesium

Magnesium is an essential mineral that accounts for about .05 percent of the body's total weight. Nearly 70 percent of the body's supply is located in the bones together with calcium and phosphorus, while 30 percent is found in soft tissues and body fluids.

Magnesium is involved in many essential metabolic processes. Most of the body's magnesium is found inside the mitochondria in the cells, where it activates enzymes necessary for the metabolism of carbohydrates and amino acids. The mitochondria accounts for nearly one third of total cellular magnesium. Magnesium is required for mitochondria energy production. Moderate magnesium deficiency is common, particularly among African Americans, and is associated with increased risks of hypertension and diabetes. By countering the stimulative effect of calcium, magnesium plays an important role in neuromuscular contraction. It also helps to regulate the acid-alkaline balance in the body.

Large amounts of magnesium can be toxic, especially if calcium intake is low and phosphorus intake is high. Excessive magnesium is usually excreted adequately, but in the event of kidney failure, there is a greater danger of toxicity because the rate of excretion is much lower.

Magnesium deficiency can occur in patients who have diabetes, pancreatitis, or kidney malfunction; are alcoholic; or consume a high-carbohydrate diet. A deficiency is related to coronary heart disease, since it results in the formation of clots in the heart and brain, and may contribute to calcium deposits. The symptoms include apprehensiveness, muscle twitching, tremors, confusion, and disorientation.

Selenium

Selenium is an essential mineral found in minute amounts in the body. It works closely with vitamin E in some of its metabolic actions, and in the promotion of normal body growth and fertility. Selenium is a natural antioxidant and appears to preserve the elasticity of tissue by delaying the oxidation of polyunsaturated fatty acids, which can cause solidification of tissue proteins.

Selenium is found in the bran and germ of cereals; in vegetables such as broccoli, onion, and tomatoes; and in tuna. The liver and kidneys contain four to five times as much selenium as do the muscles and other tissues. Selenium is normally excreted in the urine. Its presence in the feces is an indication of improper absorption.

The RDA for selenium for adults is extremely minute—five to ten parts of selenium per one million parts of food or other minerals is considered toxic. This is due to the tendency of selenium to replace sulfur in biological compounds and to inhibit the action of some enzymes. Selenium can be toxic in its pure form, so supplements should be taken with care. Reported instances of toxicity have occurred in areas where the selenium content of the soil is high. And while low doses of selenium are considered useful in preventing cataracts, higher doses have actually been found to induce cataracts. Several reports have shown selenium deficiency to cause defects in mitochondrial structure, integrity, and electron transport chain function. An increased risk of cancer and decreased immune system functioning have been associated with selenium deficiency.

A deficiency of selenium may encourage premature aging because selenium preserves tissue elasticity. This fact is of major significance for the lens within the eye, which becomes less flexible with age.

Sodium

Sodium is an essential mineral found predominantly in extracellular fluids, such as the vascular fluids within the blood vessels and the interstitial fluids surrounding the cells. The remaining sodium in the body is found within bones.

Sodium is found in virtually all foods, especially in sodium chloride (table salt). High concentrations are found in seafood, carrots, beets, poultry, and meat. Kelp is an excellent source of sodium.
There is no established dietary requirement for sodium, but it is generally observed that the usual intake far exceeds the need. The average American ingests 3 to 7 grams of sodium and 6 to 18 grams of sodium chloride each day. The NRC recommends a daily sodium-chloride intake of 1 gram for every 1 kilogram (35 ounces) of water consumed.

An excess of sodium in the diet may cause potassium to be lost in the urine. Abnormal fluid retention accompanied by dizziness and swelling of the legs or face may also occur. A daily intake of 14 to 28 grams of sodium chloride is considered excessive. Diets containing excessive amounts of sodium contribute to an increase in blood pressure. The simplest way to reduce sodium intake is to eliminate table salt from the diet.

Zinc

Zinc is an essential trace mineral that occurs in the body in a larger amount than any other trace element except iron. The human body contains approximately 1.8 grams of zinc, compared to nearly 5 grams of iron.

Zinc has a variety of functions. It is related to the normal absorption and action of the vitamins, especially vitamin A and the B complex. It is a constituent of at least twenty-five of the enzymes involved in digestion and metabolism. It is a component of insulin and part of the enzyme that is needed to break down alcohol. It also functions in carbohydrate digestion and phosphorus metabolism. It has an important role in general growth and development, proper functioning of the prostate gland, healing of wounds and burns, and synthesis of deoxyribonucleic acid (DNA).

Diets high in protein, whole-grain products, brewer's yeast, wheat bran, wheat germ, and pumpkin seeds are usually high in zinc. The RDA for zinc is 15 milligrams a day for adults. An additional 15 milligrams is recommended during pregnancy, and an additional 25 milligrams is recommended during lactation. Zinc is relatively nontoxic, although poisoning may result from eating a food that has been stored in a galvanized container. High intakes of zinc interfere with copper utilization, causing incomplete iron metabolism. When zinc is added to the diet, vitamin A is also needed in larger amounts.

Many supplements use the zinc oxide form to incorporate into their formulas. Unfortunately, this is the least biologically active form of zinc and must be combined with the proper balance of copper to avoid severe reaction. Monomethionine zinc is the most bioavailable form of zinc and the only form that does not interfere with copper absorption.

YOUR GUIDE TO MICRONUTRIENT INTAKE

While there is no "silver bullet" nutrient to solve the issues surrounding eyestrain, there are nutrients that can help to support the eye muscles, the focusing ability and coordination of the eyes, as well as the ability of the eyes to pay attention to reading material. This section will offer a listing of some of these nutrients and the food sources that are available to access the right combination of nutrients.

We should hope to get an adequate amount of nutrients from the foods we eat, but the standard American diet, appropriately abbreviated to "SAD," is woefully lacking in the proper balance of nutrients. An unbalanced diet—having too much sugar, not enough vegetables—can lead to an array of difficulties in maintaining functional visual abilities. Therefore, supplementing the diet with vitamins and minerals can be an excellent way to keep your vision strong.

	Table 9.1. Guide to Micronutrient Intake, Sources, and Benefits in Eyestrain Prevention		
Micronutrient	Recommended Daily Intake (Minimum)*	Best Sources	Benefits in Eyestrain Prevention
Vitamin A	700–900 mcg RAE**	Dairy products, liver, fish oils, leafy green vegetables, orange and yellow vegetables, tomato products, fruits	Keeps the cornea surface moist so tears can spread evenly
Vitamin B$_1$ (Thiamin)	1.1–1.2 mg	Whole grains, cereal, pasta, rice, meat (especially pork) and fish, legumes (such as black beans and soybeans), seeds, and nuts	Maintains muscle strength and concentration
Vitamin B$_2$ (Riboflavin)	1.1–1.3 mg	Eggs, organ meats (such as kidney and liver), lean meats, low-fat milk, and green vegetables such as asparagus, broccoli, and spinach	Maintains energy and concentration
Vitamin B$_5$ (Pantothenic Acid)	5 mg	Beef, poultry, seafood, organ meats, eggs, milk, whole grains, peanuts, sunflower seeds, chickpeas, and vegetables such as mushrooms, avocados, potatoes, and broccoli	Supports alertness and muscle tone
Vitamin B$_6$ (Pyridoxine)	1.3–1.7 mg	Poultry, fish, organ meats, potatoes and other starchy vegetables, fruit (other than citrus)	Important to blinking reflex, drives the conversion of omega-6 fatty acids to form PGE1
Vitamin B$_{12}$ (Cyanocobalamin)	2.4 mcg	All animal-based foods (beef, chicken, fish), no plant sources	Maintains energy levels
Choline	425–550 mg	Meat, eggs, poultry, fish, dairy, Brussels sprouts, broccoli, cauliflower, beans, nuts, seeds, and whole grains	Regulates memory, mood, and muscle control, improves cognitive functioning

Micronutrient	Recommended Daily Intake (Minimum)*	Best Sources	Benefits in Eyestrain Prevention
Vitamin C	75–90 mg	Oranges, grapefruit, red and green peppers, kiwifruit, broccoli, strawberries, cantaloupe, baked potatoes, tomatoes	Supports proper retinal functioning and lens clarity, is an antioxidant
Vitamin D₃	600–800 IU	Fatty fish such as salmon, tuna, and mackerel, and beef liver, cheese, and egg yolks.	Supports muscle tone, increases efficiency of nerves
Vitamin E	15 mg (up to 1,000 mg)	Vegetable oils such as wheat germ, sunflower, safflower, and soybean, nuts, seeds, and green vegetables such as spinach and broccoli	Supports proper retinal functioning and lens clarity, is an antioxidant that protects other nutrients
Acetyl-L-Carnitine	500 mg three times a day	Made by the body using amino acids	Supports proper brain functioning, muscle movement, and many other body processes
Alpha-Lipoic Acid	200 mg	Yeast, liver, kidney, spinach, broccoli, and potatoes	Excellent antioxidant, important for energy production, especially in diabetics
Astaxanthin	6 mg	Krill, salmon, algae, and most red-colored aquatic organisms	Supports proper muscle functioning, increases blood flow to retina
Beta-Carotene	2,000 mg	Yellow or orange fruits such as cantaloupes, mangoes, pumpkins, papayas, carrots, and sweet potatoes	Is converted into vitamin A, which supports proper retinal functioning
Cannabidiol (CBD)	No data available	Hemp	Calming effect on the nervous system, receptors in the retina, and the optic nerve
Co-Enzyme Q₁₀	25–100 mg	Created internally or taken in supplement form	Supports muscle tissue, is an antioxidant

Micronutrient	Recommended Daily Intake (Minimum)*	Best Sources	Benefits in Eyestrain Prevention
Lutein	10–20 mg	Kale, spinach, chard, egg yolks, and dark, leafy greens	Absorbs high-energy blue light in the retina, increases contrast, protects the retina and lens
Zeaxanthin	4–8 mg	Goji berries, red chili peppers, saffron, corn (non-GMO), and egg yolks	Protects the retina from blue light, increases contrast, is an antioxidant
Calcium	1,000–1,200 mg	Yogurt, cheese, sardines, salmon, soy products, and kale	Regulates the contraction of muscles, nerve conduction, and the clotting of blood
Iron	10 mg. Should be balanced with zinc intake. Consult a physician for specific recommendations	Lean meat, seafood, poultry, white beans, lentils, spinach, kidney beans, peas, nuts, and raisins.	Important for energy production and alertness.
Magnesium	350–400 mg	Pumpkin seed kernels, almonds, spinach, cashews, and peanuts	Important for muscle and nerve functioning
Selenium	55 mcg	Oysters, Brazil nuts, halibut, yellowfin tuna, eggs, sardines, sunflower seeds, chicken breast, and shiitake mushrooms	Powerful antioxidant; caution not to overdose
Sodium	1.5 mg (maximum)	Pickled preserves and jerky, processed foods, and salt	Balanced with potassium, maintains normal blood pressure and cellular health
Zinc (gluconate or acetate)	25 mg	Meat, fish, shellfish, fowl, eggs, and dairy	Mobilizes vitamin A for retinal health

* Consult your primary care provider for dosages specific to your needs.

** 900 mcg RAE is equivalent to about 3,000 IU.

CONCLUSION

Eyestrain can have many different possible causes, but nutrition is often overlooked as one of them. As you read this chapter, you might have noticed that many of the nutrients mentioned depend on other nutrients to perform their functions appropriately. Maintaining healthy eyes involves support of many nerves, blood vessels, muscles, tendons, ligaments, and a whole host of other tissues important to the visual system. As you can see, the nutrients you consume with every meal play an important role in fostering the health of every organ in your body. By being deficient in one or two key nutrients, you may end up facing a number of health-related problems, including various eye-related disorders. By understanding what your body needs, you can avoid, reduce, or eliminate such outcomes.

A lack of specific nutrients, however, is just one of the factors involved in that which you consume each day. Many people need to take various prescribed medications for a wide variety of reasons. These drugs can come with side effects that include eye-related problems. The next chapter discusses some of the side effects of certain medications that can affect the way you see and might create stress on your eyes and vision. Most medications have side effects, and talking about them with your doctor may lead to adjustments in medication dosages in order to reduce eyestrain issues.

10

Medications

As we age, we are more likely to develop a variety of different ailments. Where the general medical model is concerned, this means taking more medications. In fact, nearly one in three older adults uses multiple prescription drugs. Before taking two or more medications, always make sure that the medications you may be taking do not create a negative interaction.

Unfortunately, a medication may have side effects—in other words, effects, whether positive or negative, which are secondary to the drug's intended effect. Although the term "side effects" most often describes adverse effects, it can also apply to beneficial but unintended consequences of the use of a drug. Given that the eye has such an abundance of blood vessels, muscles, nerves, and fluids, it is more than likely that a medication prescribed for any number of medical conditions can and will affect the eyes.

Before taking any medication or medications, you should always ask your doctor or pharmacist about side effects or negative interactions with the eyes or visual system. Now let us look at some of the more commonly prescribed drugs and see how they might affect the eye. If you regularly take any of these medications and notice any of the following side effects, notify your healthcare provider as soon as possible.

Table 10.1. Common Medications and Their Ocular Side Effects

Brand Name	Generic Name	Indications	Ocular Side Effects
Accutane	Isotretinoin	Difficult cases of cystic acne, keratinization disorders, folliculitis, psoriasis	Redness, dry eye, corneal opacities, tearing, optic neuritis, light sensitivity, floaters, contact-lens intolerance, night blindness

Brand Name	Generic Name	Indications	Ocular Side Effects
Achromycin	Tetracycline	Acne, chlamydia	Retinal hemorrhage, decreased vision, headaches, light sensitivity, nearsightedness, enlarged blind spot
Actifed	Pseudoephedrine	Allergic rhinitis, allergic conjunctivitis, motion sickness	Hallucinations, decreased eye pressure, dilated pupils, dry eye
Aricept	Donepezil	Alzheimer's disease	Cataracts, glaucoma, retinal hemorrhages, conjunctival hemorrhages, eye irritation, blepharitis, dry eye, floaters
Arimidex	Anastrozole	Breast cancer	Cataracts
Atrovent	Ipratropium bromide	Rhinitis	Worsened narrow-angle glaucoma, pink eye, dry eye, blurred vision, eye pain
Benadryl	Diphenhydramine	Allergic rhinitis, allergic conjunctivitis, motion sickness	Visual-field constriction, hallucinations, retinal hemorrhages
Betoptic	Betaxolol	Open-angle glaucoma	Hallucinations, decreased tear flow (dry eye), redness, double vision, drooping eyelids
Cafergot	Ergotamine	Migraine	Spasms and constriction of blood vessels in all parts of the eye
Cardizem	Diltiazem	Angina due to coronary artery spasm, mild to moderate hypertension	Pain, redness, dizziness, hallucinations, tearing, eye irritation
Catapres	Clonidine	Hypertension	Eye irritation, dry eyes, hallucinations, dilated pupils
Coumadin	Warfarin sodium	Venous thrombosis, atrial fibrillation with embolization, pulmonary emboli, coronary occlusion	Tearing, cataracts, hemorrhages, decreased vision, yellowing of eyes
Desyrel	Trazodone	Depression	Optic neuritis, lazy eye, retinal or subconjunctival hemorrhages, light sensitivity, dry eye, decreased vision

Brand Name	Generic Name	Indications	Ocular Side Effects
Detrol	Tolterodine tartrate	Bladder control problems	Headaches, dry eye, hallucinations, blurred near vision, glaucoma
Diabinese	Chlorpropamide	Diabetes	Optic neuritis, yellowing eyes, disturbed color vision, retinal hemorrhages, light sensitivity, double vision
Dilantin	Phenytoin	Epilepsy	Retinal hemorrhages, nystagmus, yellowing of eyes, double vision, disturbed accommodation, flashing lights, glare sensitivity, disturbed color vision
Dimetapp	Brompheniramine	Cough and upper respiratory symptoms, including nasal congestion, associated with allergy or common cold	Different size pupils, visual-field constriction, hallucinations, dry eye, double vision
Diuril	Chlorothiazide	Hypertension, edema associated with congestive heart failure, cirrhosis, corticosteroid or estrogen therapy	Edema, retinal hemorrhages, disturbed accommodation, nearsightedness, yellow vision
Donnatal	Phenobarbital	Epilepsy, anxiety	Blind spots, hallucinations, lazy eye, optic neuritis, involuntary eye movements, blurred vision, pupil dilation
Elavil	Amitriptyline	Depression	Hallucinations, retinal hemorrhages, lazy eye, optic neuritis, dry eye, yellowing, increased eye pressure
Enduron	Methyclothiazide	Hypertension, edema associated with congestive heart failure, cirrhosis, premenstrual tension, corticosteroid or estrogen therapy.	Edema, retinal hemorrhages, decreased vision, disturbed accommodation, redness, light sensitivity

Brand Name	Generic Name	Indications	Ocular Side Effects
Fosamax	Alendronate sodium	Osteoporosis	Inflammation of the sclera, uveitis
Humulin	Insulin	Diabetes	Decreased pupil reaction, double vision, involuntary eye movements, blurred vision.
Imitrex	Sumatriptan	Migraine	Eye muscle weakness, accommodative disorder, dilated pupils, ocular hemorrhages, eye pain, double vision, conjunctivitis, ocular edema, corneal opacities
Inderal	Propranolol	Hypertension	Drooping eyelids, double vision, decreased vision, hallucinations, dry eye, headache
Ismelin	Guanethidine	Hypertension	Light sensitivity, burning, double vision, accommodative spasm, flashing lights
Lamictal	Lomtrigine	Seizures	Dizziness, ataxia, sedation, involuntary eye movements, blurred vision, double vision
Lanoxin	Digoxin	Congestive heart failure, atrial fibrillation or flutter, atrial tachycardia	Optic neuritis, disturbed color vision, blurred vision, headache, yellow vision, hallucinations, glare sensitivity, halos around lights, double vision
Lasix	Furosemide	Hypertension	Blurred vision, dizziness, headache
Librium	Chlordiazepoxide	Anxiety	Disturbed depth perception, retinal hemorrhage, disturbed accommodation, yellowing of eye
Lipitor	Atorvastatin	Elevated cholesterol	Swelling around eyelids, red eyes, itchiness, myasthenia gravis, headache, light sensitivity
Lithobid	Lithium	Manic phase of bipolar disorder	Blind spots, retinal or subconjunctival hemorrhages, hallucinations, light sensitivity, involuntary eye movements, dry eye

Brand Name	Generic Name	Indications	Ocular Side Effects
Mellaril	Thioridazine	Psychosis	Night blindness, blind spots, cataracts, blurred vision, hallucinations, lazy eye, crossed eyes, light sensitivity, yellowing, optic atrophy, discolored eyes
Mevacor	Lovastatin	Elevated cholesterol	Cataracts, blurred vision, headache
Motrin	Ibuprofen	Osteoarthritis, pain, fever	Blind spots, visual-field constriction, lazy eye, retinal hemorrhages, optic neuritis, dry eyes
Niaspan	Niacin	Elevated cholesterol	Blurred vision, lazy eye, central blind spot, glaucoma, protruding eyes
Norpramin	Desipramine	Depression	Hallucinations, lazy eye, optic neuritis, dryness, blurred vision, headache, light sensitivity, yellowing of the eyes, disturbed accommodation
Norvasc	Amlodipine	Hypertension, angina	Blurred vision, headache, vertigo, visual distortion, yellowing
Ortho-Novum	Norethindrone	Birth control	Optic neuritis, blind spots, halos around lights, cataracts, headache, yellowing of eyes
Orudis	Ketoprofen	Rheumatoid arthritis	Decreased vision, retinal or subconjunctival hemorrhages, eye pain, hallucinations, visual-field constriction, pink eye
Paxil	Paroxetine hydrochloride	Depression	Dry eye, abnormal vision, blurred vision, headache, dizziness
Pepcid	Famotidine	Duodenal ulcer, benign gastric ulcer	Decreased vision, hallucinations, retinal or subconjunctival hemorrhages, light sensitivity, yellowing

Brand Name	Generic Name	Indications	Ocular Side Effects
Plaquenil	Hydroxychloroquine	Malaria, rheumatoid arthritis, lupus erythematosus	Cataracts, eye pigmentation, focusing difficulty, eye blisters, eye-muscle paralysis, accommodative difficulty, halos around lights, hallucinations, night blindness, flashing lights
Pravachol	Pravastatin sodium	Elevated cholesterol	Headache, muscle weakness, dizziness
Premarin	Estrogen	Menopause, osteoporosis, female hypogonadism, atrophic vaginitis, breast cancer, prostate cancer	Optic neuritis, blind spots, disturbed color vision, yellowing of eyes, nearsightedness, dry eye, fluctuations in vision, contact-lens intolerance
Prozac	Fluoxetine	Depression	Pain, light sensitivity, dry eye, iritis, cataracts, double vision, drooping eyelids
Restoril	Temazepam	Insomnia, anxiety, tension, agitation, skeletal-muscle spasms	Pain, disturbed accommodation, yellowing, hallucinations, tearing, burning, light sensitivity, nystagmus
Retin-A	Tretinoin	Acne	Skin dryness, light sensitivity, red eyes, red eyelids
Ritalin	Methylphenidate	Attention deficit hyperactivity disorder	Retinal or subconjunctival hemorrhages, dilated pupils, hallucinations, blurred vision, redness
Rogaine	Minoxidil	Hair loss	Increased eye pressure, decreased vision, optic neuritis, blurred vision
Synthroid	Levothyroxine	Hypothyroidism	Decreased vision, double vision, drooping eyelids, yellow eyes, dry eye
Tagamet	Cimetidine	Ulcers	Hallucinations, light sensitivity, blurred vision, redness, irritation/dryness
Tavist	Clemastine	Mild allergy symptoms	Decreased vision, dryness, light sensitivity, eyelid swelling, hallucinations, different-sized pupils

Brand Name	Generic Name	Indications	Ocular Side Effects
Tenormin	Atenolol	Hypertension	Decreased vision, hallucinations, dry eye, burning, redness, yellow eyes
Timoptic	Timolol maleate	Glaucoma	Dryness, burning, blurred vision, pupil size variations, droopy eyelids, nearsightedness, hallucinations
Topamax	Topiramate	Seizures	Glaucoma, increase tearing, double vision, myopia
Tylenol	Acetaminophen	Fever, mild pain	Hallucinations, disturbed color vision, double vision, redness
Viagra	Sildenafil	Erectile dysfunction	Blurred vision, yellow vision, sensitivity to light, blue vision, double vision, hemorrhages, burning eyes
Voltaren	Diclofenac	Rheumatoid arthritis, osteoarthritis, post-eye surgery.	Blurred vision, night blindness, lazy eye, blind spots, bleeding in the eye, itchiness, tearing, light sensitivity
Xanax	Alprazolam	Anxiety, depression	Disturbed color vision, disturbed accommodation, pain, hallucinations, uncontrolled eye movements, yellow eyes
Zestril	Ace Inhibitor	Hypertension	Yellow eyes, dizziness, headache
Zantac	Ranitidine	Gastric ulcers	Disturbed color vision, hallucinations, blurred vision, eyelid swelling, yellowing, redness
Zocor	Simvastatin	Elevated cholesterol	Blurred vision, worsened cataracts, eye-muscle weakness
Zoloft	Sertaline	Depression	Eye pain, blind spots, dry eye, light sensitivity, double vision, increased tearing
Zyrtec	Cetirizine	Allergies	Ocular melanoma, glaucoma, ocular hemorrhage, loss of accommodation, dryness, headache, loss of visual field

CONCLUSION

As you can see, just about every medication you are likely to take can have some effect on the eyes or visual system. Remember that these drugs are prescribed because the main effect is more beneficial than any side effects. You only have one set of eyes, though, so it is important to consider the effect of medications on them as well. Again, always check with your physician or pharmacist if you have any questions or concerns regarding visual effects of any medications you are taking. Lastly, and just as important, should you experience a side effect or negative interaction with any drug you happen to be taking, contact your doctor, who may be able to prescribe an alternative medication that does not come with these issues.

Lifestyle can also affect eye performance and ocular health. Smoking, pollution, lack of exercise, poor dietary habits, and excessive work pressure are just some of the factors that can lead to eyestrain and a poorly performing visual system. The next chapter offers techniques that can assist in the relaxation of the eyes, ensuring clear and comfortable vision in a variety of circumstances.

11

Eye Exercises

Eyestrain is typically a reaction of the eyes to stressful situations, whether those situations are due to poor lighting, poor nutrition, or simply part of the normal aging process. In most viewing situations, the eyes must overcome some imperfect conditions. Making sure that the eyes are functioning to their optimal level is critical to comfortable seeing. This chapter describes various eye exercises, which, if performed on a regular basis, may help the eyes to work with ease.

Like many parts of the body, the eyes are dependent on muscles to maneuver and position themselves in the optimum spot in order to be effective. It is obviously more challenging when there are two eyes (nature usually provides for a spare organ in case of failure) that need to move in coordinated effort with each other. One might think that muscle strength is the most important factor in the achievement of comfortable sight. Coordination between the two eyes, not just strength, however, plays more of a crucial role in how we see.

YOUR EYE MUSCLES

There are six eye muscles around the outside of each eyeball, known as extraocular muscles. These muscles are called striated muscles and are similar to the more commonly known biceps and triceps of the arms. This type of muscle tissue contains fibrils in the cells, which are aligned in parallel bundles so that their different regions form stripes. Muscles of this kind are often attached to the skeleton by tendons and are under voluntary control. This is actually true for the eyes as well, since they are anchored to the skull at the back of the eye socket. These eye muscles are about 200 times as strong as they need to be to move an eyeball. Thus, when someone refers to a "weak" eye, it is rarely a defect in the muscle that is causing this concern.

Within the eye, there are muscles that control the size of the pupil, which is actually a hole in the colored iris. Therefore, the muscles in the iris are smooth muscles and are not under voluntary control. These two sets of muscles either dilate (expand) the pupil or constrict (shrink) the pupil. The size of the pupil is important in controlling the amount of light entering the eye, as well as creating a sharper image on the retina. One reason we see less accurately at night is that the pupil must remain

Optometric Vision Therapy

Optometric vision therapy combines a series of office visits with exercises done at home. "Exercise," in this case, does not refer to aerobic exercise or strength training, but rather to activities designed to improve binocular coordination and eye-brain coordination. When you practice vision exercises or techniques, you will not strengthen your eye muscles (they are already strong enough), but you will improve the efficiency and smoothness of the muscles that control your eye movements and the focusing of your eyes' lenses. You will also improve the connections between your eyes and your brain, and between your two eyes. Some of the visual skills that optometric vision therapy seeks to improve are:

- **Accommodation:** the ability to look quickly from far to near and vice versa, such as from the dashboard to the cars on the street, or from the chalkboard to a book, without blurriness.

- **Attention maintenance:** the ability to continue doing a particular skill or activity with ease and without interfering with the performance of other skills.

- **Binocular coordination:** the ability to use both eyes together, smoothly, equally, simultaneously, and accurately.

- **Depth perception:** the ability to judge the relative distances of objects, and to see and move accurately within a three-dimensional space, such as when parking a car.

dilated at this time, allowing as much of the small amount of available light at night to enter the eye, but this dilation also increases the optical distortion that blurs the image.

Another muscle within the eye is called the ciliary muscle. This is a circular muscle surrounding and attached to the crystalline lens. When this muscle contracts, the diameter of the muscle gets smaller, allowing the crystalline lens to expand, thus creating more focusing power. So, when looking at a near object (within twenty feet), the ciliary muscle constricts and allows the near object to maintain a clear image on the retina. This process allows us to see clearly at both far and near

- **Distance-vision acuity:** the ability to see, inspect, identify, and interpret objects clearly at a distance (more than twenty feet away from the eyes).

- **Fixation:** the ability to quickly and accurately locate and inspect with both eyes a series of stationary objects, one after another, such as the words in a sentence while reading.

- **Hand-eye coordination:** the ability to use the hands and eyes together in a synchronized manner so that a task such as hitting a ball can be performed with efficiency.

- **Near-vision acuity:** the ability to see, inspect, identify, and interpret objects clearly at near distances (within twenty feet of the eyes).

- **Peripheral vision:** the ability to monitor and interpret what is happening around you while attending to a specific task with your central vision, the ability to use visual information perceived from a large area.

- **Relaxation:** the ability to relax the eyes and the visual system. This is important in the prevention and treatment of eyestrain.

- **Tracking:** the ability to follow a moving object, such as a ball in flight or vehicles in traffic, smoothly and accurately with both eyes.

- **Visualization:** the ability to form mental images in the "mind's eye" and retain them for future recall or for synthesis into new mental images beyond the current or past experiences.

distances. While it seems that you can actively control this action, this muscle is governed by the parasympathetic nervous system, which is not typically under voluntary control.

There are two neurological systems that control the movement of the eyes. One deals with convergence, which controls the aiming of the eyes to maintain single vision. The other deals with focusing and activates the lens to maintain a clear image. These two systems are coordinated in the brain. Thus, as recently explained, when there is a "lazy eye" or a "wandering eye," a weak muscle is rarely the cause of the problem. The fault lies in the coordination centers within the brain. The ability to train these actions, however, is possible with vision therapy.

There are several techniques that can be used to retrain the eyes and visual system when poor coordination occurs. Given that there are so many types of eye disorders that can arise, it is difficult to say exactly which technique would be the proper one to enhance your particular visual deficiency. Functional vision optometrists (also called behavioral vision optometrists), however, specialize in this area, and have had tremendous success in resolving many of these types of vision concerns. The techniques included here can enhance the general visual abilities of most individuals with the most common concerns related to eyestrain.

Only a professional evaluation from the proper eyecare specialist will be able to confirm which techniques are most appropriate. In addition, these are self-directed techniques, whereas professional office procedures use other instrumentation that might be more effective and faster acting to resolve visual concerns. A listing of the appropriate organizations to find one of these specialists is listed in the Resources section (see page 167) at the end of this book.

VISION THERAPY TECHNIQUES

Vision therapy techniques can improve the skills just mentioned in the previous index. The following are some techniques that are similar to what you can do at a doctor's office but adapted so you can do them at home. The goal of vision therapy is to increase the person's visual abilities so that reading and other visually intensive tasks can be performed with less effort and thus less eyestrain. It is usually best to do these techniques early in the day, before your eyes are too tired. Do not try to do all these techniques every day. Instead, spread them over the course of a few days. If some of these are difficult at first, do not be concerned. As you continue to perform these tasks regularly, you will find them easier to do as your visual system performance improves.

Accommodative Rock

This technique helps to improve the eyes' ability to change focus and see clearly at near and at distance. Accommodation is the process by which the eyes change focus, and is probably the most important and most often performed function of the eyes. The ability to focus decreases with age, but adequate focusing ability can be maintained for longer periods with techniques such as this one. To do the accommodative rock:

1. Fasten some large letters, such as a banner newspaper headline, to a wall, and stand back twenty feet. If necessary, use your glasses to see the letters clearly.

2. Take some small letters, such as the body of a newspaper article, and hold them in one hand.

3. Cover one of your eyes with your free hand, keeping the eye itself open, and bring the small print as close to your face as you can while still being able to see it clearly. Stop.

4. Look at the large letters on the wall again. Are they clear?

5. Continuing to hold the small print at the same distance, look at it again. Is it clear?

6. Repeat steps 4 and 5 for a few minutes until you can see both the distance and near letters easily. The accommodation should take only a second. Try the technique with the other eye, and then repeat it with the small letters held one-inch closer.

Do this technique for five minutes with each eye at least twice a day. Preferably, finish both sessions before evening tiredness sets in. You can also try this technique throughout the day, whenever you find yourself with a near and a distant object on which to focus—for example, a wall clock and your wristwatch.

Rotations

Rotations increase the eyes' tracking ability and help your ability to pay attention to an activity. Smooth eye movements are basic to good vision. You will need an empty pie pan and a marble for this technique. To do rotations:

1. Put the marble in the pie pan and hold the pie pan about sixteen inches from your eyes.

2. Tilt the pie tin so that the marble rolls around the edge at a steady pace. Follow the marble with your eyes only; do not move your head.

3. Repeat step 2, rolling the marble around the edge of the pie pan in the opposite direction.

Do this technique for two minutes in each direction once a day. (You can become dizzy if you keep the marble going in the same direction for more than two minutes). If possible, have a friend watch your eyes to see how smoothly they move.

Alphabet Fixations

Alphabet fixations improve the ability to center the eyes—that is, to fixate them—on an object in an instant. Fixation is one of the skills used in reading. This technique also helps with near-vision acuity. To do alphabet fixations:

1. Cut two strips of paper. Type or clearly print the alphabet in a vertical direction on each strip.

2. Hold the strips about eighteen inches from your face and a bit farther apart than shoulder width.

3. Call out the letters in alphabetical order, making sure to read each letter off a strip before calling out its name. Alternate between the strips, reading the "a" from one strip, the "b" from the second, the "c" from the first strip again, and so on. Keep your head absolutely still as you do this.

4. Spell words using the strips, again reading the letters before calling them out and alternating between the two strips as in step 3. For

example, spell the word "boy" by taking the "b" from the left-hand strip, the "o" from the right-hand strip, and the "y" from the left-hand strip again. Your speed should increase with practice.

Do this technique for five minutes once a day.

Monocular Fixations

The monocular (one-eyed) fixation technique enhances the ability to fixate with one eye at a time. This particular technique can improve hand-eye coordination. You will need a string, a small ring (such as a wedding band or a key ring), and a knitting needle or long pencil. To do monocular fixations:

1. Tie the string to the ring and hang the string (from a doorway, for example) so that the ring is at eye level. Stand about two feet away from the ring.

2. Hold the knitting needle or pencil in your right hand, cover your left eye, step forward on your right foot, and try to put the knitting needle or pencil through the ring without touching it. Try this several times.

3. Move the knitting needle or pencil to your left hand, cover your right eye, step forward on your left foot, and try to put the knitting needle or pencil through the ring again without touching it.

4. After mastering the technique using a stationary ring, repeat steps 2 and 3 with a swinging ring. This is great practice for many sports.

Do this technique for five minutes with each eye once a day.

Wall Fixations

Wall fixations improve your ability to fixate and your peripheral vision at the same time. You will need eight white 3x5-inch index cards, a felt-tipped marker, a blank wall, a book, and maybe some gentle music. To do wall fixations:

1. Number the index cards from one to eight, one number per card. Using the felt-tipped marker and a bold stroke, position each number

in the center of the card and make it two inches tall. Fasten the cards in a haphazard order to a blank wall in an eight-foot square. (See Figure 11.1 below.)

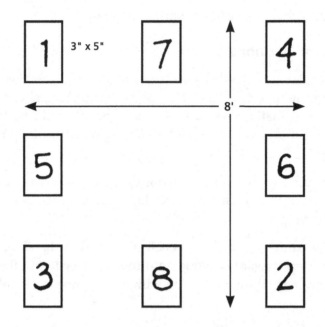

Figure 11.1. Wall Fixations

2. Stand about six feet from the wall, facing the center of the card pattern. Put a book on your head to keep your head steady, and cover one eye.

3. Starting with the "1" card, shift your eyes from card to card in numerical order. Keep your head very still and look directly at each number, being aware of the other numbers in your peripheral vision. If you wish, do this technique to gentle music to help keep your eye movements smooth and steady.

4. When you become adept at shifting your eyes from card to card, move closer to the wall. Continue to move closer as your skill improves. As you move closer to the wall, your eye movements will need to become extreme.

5. Repeat steps 3 and 4 first with the other eye, and then with both eyes together.

Do this technique for two minutes with each eye, and then for two minutes with both eyes, once a day.

Another similar solution is the "Eye Yoga" headset. It runs a five-minute gentle eye exercise program, designed to target the source of the discomfort, offering relief by encouraging the eye muscles to stretch and relax, hence increasing blood flow and nutrient distribution to these areas, improving the user's physical and mental focus, with the eye feeling rejuvenated and refreshed, and minimizing the symptoms of eyestrain. It is easy to use and safe for the whole family. (See Resources on page 167 for information on how to find the Eye Yoga device.)

Marsden Ball

The Marsden ball technique is a great activity for improving tracking and fixation, as well as hand-eye coordination and attention maintenance. You will need a rubber ball about four inches in diameter, some strong thread or string, and a ballpoint pen. To do the Marsden ball:

1. Write letters randomly all over the ball with the ballpoint pen. Attach the thread or string to the ball, and suspend the ball (from a doorway, for example) so that it can swing freely.

2. Cover one of your eyes, give the ball a slight push, and try to touch one letter at a time, calling out the letter at you do so. Keep your head as still as possible.

3. Repeat step 2 with the other eye.

Do this technique for two minutes with each eye once a day.

Deep Blink

The deep blink can improve your ability to accommodate and the acuity of your distance vision. It is also a relaxation technique. Note that if you feel dizzy or faint at any time while performing the technique, then you should stop and rest. You will need a blank wall, a chair, and some large letters, such as a banner newspaper headline. To do the deep blink:

1. Fasten the large letters to the wall and remove your glasses or contacts. Stand a few feet from the letters and gradually move back until the letters start to blur. Position the chair at this point.

2. Sit in the chair in a relaxed posture. Take a deep breath and let it out slowly. Repeat this a few times until you feel relaxed.

3. Take a deep breath and hold it. With your breath held, close your eyes, clench your fists, and tighten the muscles in your whole body—legs, arms, stomach, chest, neck, face, head, and eyes. Keep your muscles tightened for about five seconds.

4. At the end of the five seconds, snap your hands and eyes open, exhale quickly through your mouth, and relax your entire body. Breathe slowly, and look at the letters, blinking gently as necessary. Stay very relaxed and try to look through, rather than at, the letters. After a second or two, the letters should become clear. (If you feel dizzy or faint after tightening and relaxing your muscles, omit this part. Just take slow, deep breaths, and practice looking through the letters on the wall.)

5. If the letters remained clear, push your chair about a foot back from the wall, and repeat steps 3 and 4. Continue moving your chair back to see how far away you can sit from the letters and still keep them clear. You may be amazed to find that after a few weeks, you can sit quite a few feet further back from where you started and still see those letters.

Do this technique at least once a day.

Brock String Technique

The Brock string technique helps to improve depth perception, peripheral vision, and binocular coordination. You will need a piece of string four feet in length. To do the Brock string technique:

1. Tie a knot in the middle of the string. Attach one end of the string to any object that is at your eye level. (You can sit or stand for this technique.) Hold the string between your thumb and forefinger, stretch it taut, and hold it up against your nose.

2. Look at the far end of the string. You should see an A without the crossbar. You should see the knot in the middle of the string as two knots, one on each side of the A. (See Figure 11.2 below.)

3. Look at the knot in the string. It may take a few seconds, but you should be able to see an X pattern with one knot in the middle.

4. Shift your gaze back and forth from the A to the X pattern until the movement is smooth and requires little effort.

5. Move your gaze up the string toward your nose. As you do this, you should find the center of the X moving up toward your nose, too. When your gaze gets very close to your nose, the X should become a V, and the knot in the middle of the string should appear to be two knots, one on each side of the V, in your peripheral vision.

6. Shift your gaze from the A to the X to the V pattern until the movement is smooth and requires little effort. Continue shifting your gaze, shortening the string but keeping the knot centered.

Do this technique for five minutes once a day.

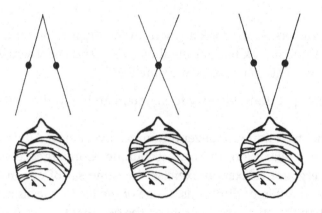

Figure 11.2. Brock String Technique

Convergence Stimulation

Convergence is the aiming of the eyes toward one another as you look at near objects. This skill is critical for all near-point activities, such as reading. Convergence stimulation helps to develop binocular coordination, of which convergence is one aspect, and good depth perception. It also improves attention maintenance. You will need Figure 11.3 on page 153 and a pencil. To do convergence stimulation:

1. Hold the illustration at your normal reading distance and focus your eyes on it. If necessary, wear your glasses or contact lenses. You should see two sets of concentric circles.

2. Position the point of the pencil in between the two sets of concentric circles and focus on it, remaining at your normal reading distance.

3. Move the pencil slowly toward your eyes, leaving the illustration where it is. Keep focusing on the point of the pencil, but be aware of the circles beyond it as you do. You should begin to see three, rather than two, sets of concentric circles when the pencil is approximately six inches from your eyes. The set in the middle (the one that is not there) should appear as a three-dimensional figure, farther away from you than the larger ones and resembling a cup or flowerpot. Keep the pencil still and keep looking at it. Your eyes should feel as if they are crossing (they are actually just pulling in toward each other).

4. Relax your focus and look away from the illustration for a second or two, and then look back at the illustration and see if you can regain the image. This may take some practice.

5. Repeat step 4 until it is easy to maintain and hold the center image.

Do this technique for several minutes every day. Alternate it with convergence relaxation, the next technique. Convergence stimulation and convergence relaxation exercise the same set of eye muscles, but pull them in different directions. If one of the techniques is much easier for you than the other, concentrate on the one that is more difficult until you can do it as easily as the other one.

Convergence Relaxation

Convergence relaxation is the opposite of convergence. It is the ability of the eyes to relax—that is, to diverge from their converged position—as they focus on a distant object. Excessive near-point work can cause the eyes to have trouble relaxing, so practicing convergence relaxation is good for breaking up your day if you do a lot of reading or computer work. The technique helps with binocular coordination, depth perception, and attention maintenance. You will once again need Figure 11.3, below, plus a blank wall. To practice convergence relaxation:

1. Stand at least ten feet away from the blank wall and focus your eyes on it.

2. Slowly bring the illustration into your line of sight at your normal reading distance, but keep your eyes focused on the wall. You can hold the illustration just above the point on the wall where your eyes are focused. You should see three sets of concentric circles, just as you did in the convergence-stimulation technique. But this time, while the center set of circles should still seem to be three-dimensional, it should also appear to be closer to you than the outside circles and resemble upside-down cups or flower pots. The other sets of circles, which will be in your peripheral vision, may appear this way, too.

3. Relax your focus and look away from the illustration for a second or two, and then look back at the illustration and see if you can regain the image. This may take some practice.

4. Repeat step 3 until it is easy to maintain and hold the center image.

Do this technique for several minutes every day. Alternate it with convergence stimulation, the previous technique.

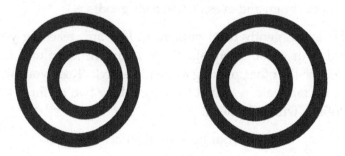

Figure 11.3. Convergence Stimulation and Convergence Relaxation

Palming

Palming is a relaxation technique to use between other techniques and throughout the day. It allows you to relax your mind and your eyes because you do not focus on anything but blackness. It can also increase your visualization skills. Palming is adapted from the *Bates method,* which is a system of techniques devised by Dr. William Bates to improve eyesight. (Dr. Bates theorized that stress is the cause of most vision problems, and that relaxation is the cure.) To do palming:

1. Close your eyes and cover them with your hands. Keep your palms over, but not touching, your eyelids. Your fingers should overlap near your hairline, and you should have enough room to breathe easily. Rest your elbows on a table. All you should see is complete blackness. If you see flashes of light, just let them go and allow the blackness to return. You can either continue to focus on the blackness, or you can now start to visualize a relaxing scene of your own choosing.

2. Take a deep breath and feel the muscles around your eyes completely relax. Breathe deeply and slowly eight times.

Do this technique as needed, at least eight times a day, preferably before you start an intense near-point task, such as reading or computer work.

Head Rolling

Head rolling is another relaxation technique based on the Bates method. It increases the blood flow, which increases the flow of life-maintaining oxygen, to the brain and eyes. It also feels good!

1. While seated, gently drop your head forward, reaching your chin toward your chest. Then, slowly roll your head around from one shoulder to the other, making a complete circle. Keep your shoulders level and maintain regular breathing. Make two or three complete revolutions with your head.

2. Repeat step 1, rolling your head in the other direction.

Do this technique first thing in the morning and again later in the afternoon for a relaxation break. It is also good to do this technique as a short break from computer work.

CONCLUSION

Remember that eye exercises are not about strengthening eye muscles but more about coordination between the two eyes, as well as the focusing system. By itself, a vision therapy program can guide you to reduce eyestrain but must be combined with a shift in lifestyle choices, including management of work stress, family issues, computer and digital screen time, and nutrition. Reducing eyestrain is easier to do before your eyes adapt to the stressors of daily life.

Conclusion

I f you are reading this book, the odds are very good that you or a loved one may be suffering from eyestrain. For some, these problems can range from mild but constant to debilitating. Over the years, I have had many patients come into my office complaining of a variety of eye problems—from headaches to red eyes to blurred vision. After asking a few questions, the majority of them seem to be suffering from the many symptoms of eyestrain. In this book, I have tried to explain the many causes of eyestrain and what you can do to lessen or eliminate these problems. By understanding the basics of these underlying issues, you can determine what you can do for yourself. Whether it is by improving your lighting, reading large-print books, or simply going to your local eye professional to have your eyes checked, you can play a major role in overcoming these symptoms.

As you can see in the Table 2.1 in Chapter 2 (see page 17), I have laid out the symptoms and possible causes. I strongly suggest that if your problem should persist you find the appropriate health professional to help you. The bottom line here is that you can control your own health more than you would imagine.

Your eyes are not only the windows to the soul, but also the mirror of the body. With just a bit of effort, you should be able resolve any eyestrain issues and maintain healthy functional eyesight throughout your lifetime.

Here's looking at you!

Glossary

accommodation. The ability of the eye to adjust its focus for near vision, distance vision, and all points in-between.

amblyopia. *See* lazy eye.

antioxidant. A substance that blocks oxidation reactions in the body, some of which can lead to cellular dysfunction and destruction. The antioxidant nutrients include beta-carotene, vitamin C, vitamin E, and selenium. Other antioxidants are the amino acid glutathione, and the enzymes superoxide dismutase (SOD), peroxidase, and catalase.

aqueous humor. A watery fluid that surrounds the iris and lens in the front part of the eye and provides some nutrition to the adjoining parts of the eye. Also called the aqueous fluid.

asthenopia. The medical term for eyestrain.

astigmatism. A condition in which the cornea is shaped more like the side of a barrel than the side of a ball, causing the light passing through it to be spread over a diffuse area of the retina rather than focused into a single point; a refractive error. *See also* emmetropia; farsightedness; nearsightedness; presbyopia; refractive error.

Bates method. A system of techniques devised by Dr. William Bates to improve eyesight. Dr. Bates theorized that stress is the cause of most vision problems, and that relaxation is the cure.

beta-carotene. A nutrient related to vitamin A that is used by the body to manufacture vitamin A. Beta-carotene is an excellent antioxidant.

bifocal lens. A corrective lens that contains two segments—one for distance viewing and one for near viewing. *See also* lens; trifocal lens.

binocular. Two-eyed.

binocular coordination. The ability to use both eyes in a smooth, efficient manner.

bioflavonoids. A diverse group of compounds found in most plants, including fruits and vegetables. They can act as antioxidants, immune-system regulators, and anti-inflammatory agents.

blue light. Light with a wavelength of between 400 and 500 nanometers. It can cause damage to the retina.

carbohydrates. Nutrients that are the main source of blood glucose, supplying the body with the energy it needs to function.

carotenoid. A yellow, orange, or red fat-soluble pigment that gives color to plants, acts as an antioxidant, and may be converted into vitamin A.

cataract. A condition in which the lens inside the eye loses its transparency and begins to become opaque, eventually preventing light from reaching the retina. *See also* congenital cataract; glass blower's cataract; secondary cataract; senile cataract.

chalazion. A condition in which the duct of one of the meibomian glands in the eyelid becomes plugged, resulting in inflammation. Also called a meibomian cyst. *See also* stye.

choroid. A layer between the retina and sclera, consisting primarily of blood vessels that provide nourishment to the retina.

ciliary muscle. A muscle that controls the focusing of the lens.

color receptors. *See* cones.

computer vision syndrome. The complex of eye and vision problems associated with near work that are experienced during or after computer work. *See also* digital eyestrain.

cones. The specialized, cone-shaped cells in the retina of the eye. They are responsible for color vision. Also called color receptors. *See also* photoreceptors; rods.

conjunctivitis. *See* pink eye.

contact lens. An artificial lens that rests on the cornea of the eye, and corrects for refractive errors. *See also* bifocal contact lens; daily-wear contact lens; disposable contact lens; extended-wear contact lens;

flexible-wear contact lens; gas-permeable contact lens; hard contact lens; lens; rigid gas-permeable contact lens.

convergence. The moving of the two eyes toward each other. This normally happens when the eyes change focus from distance to near.

convergence insufficiency. A condition in which the line of sight of both eyes don't turn in far enough when viewing a near object.

cornea. The outermost, transparent part of the outer protective layer of the eye. Its bulging curvature is responsible for most of the refraction that occurs in the eye.

CR-39. A type of plastic material used to make eyeglass lenses.

crossed eyes. A condition in which one eye turns inward while the other eye looks straight ahead. *See also* strabismus; walleyed.

cystoid maculopathy. A condition in which the macula of the retina swells, causing visual distortions.

depth perception. The ability to perceive size and distance relationships among objects in space.

deuteranopia. A defect in the perception of the color green. *See also* protanopia.

digital eyestrain. Eyestrain that results from the use of a digital viewing screen.

diplopia. *See* double vison.

distance-vision acuity. The ability to see objects twenty or more feet away.

double vision. The condition of seeing double. Also called diplopia.

dry eye disease. A condition in which the tear film of the eye is deficient or evaporates too quickly.

dyslexia. An inability to read and understand written language despite having normal intelligence.

emmetropia. The condition of the optically normal eye. When light passes through the cornea, it comes to a focus directly on the retina. *See also* astigmatism; farsightedness; nearsightedness; presbyopia; refractive error.

ergonomics. The study of people in their work environment, which is performed in an effort to prevent injury or discomfort due to the makeup of their work environments.

esotropia. Form of strabismus in which one eye turns in. *See also* strabismus.

exotropia. Form of strabismus in which one eye turns out. *See also* strabismus.

extraocular muscles. The muscles outside the eyeball that control eye movement.

farsightedness. A condition in which the eye is too short or the cornea too flat, causing the light passing through the cornea to come to a focus behind the retina when viewing a distant object; a refractive error. The farsighted person can see distant objects clearly, but sees near objects as blurry. Also called hyperopia. *See also* astigmatism; emmetropia; nearsightedness; presbyopia; refractive error.

fat. A nutrient composed of building blocks called fatty acids. It is the most concentrated source of energy available to the body.

focusing flexibility. The ability of the eye to easily change its focusing power from distance to near to distance again.

fovea. The central part of the macula.

free radicals. Molecules that easily react with other molecules and can lead to oxidative damage in the body.

hand-eye coordination. The ability to use the eyes and hands together to accomplish a task.

hyperopia. *See* farsightedness.

iris. The colored portion of the eye that surrounds the pupil. Its expansion decreases the amount of light entering the eye through the pupil, and its contraction increases the amount of light.

keratoconus. A condition in which the cornea has a cone-like bulge.

lactoferrin. A protein found in tears that helps the eye to maintain a moist surface.

lazy eye. A condition in which a healthy eye cannot achieve 20/20 vision with any corrective device. It usually results from the brain suppressing the vision in that eye to avoid seeing two different images from the two eyes. Also called amblyopia.

lens. The resilient, transparent structure in the eye that focuses light on the retina by changing the curvature of its front surface. It is located near the front of the eye, directly behind the pupil. Also, a transparent device that corrects for refractive errors by causing light to be focused on the retina of the eye. It includes eyeglass lenses, contact lenses, and the artificial intraocular lenses that are implanted after cataract surgery. *See also* artificial intraocular lens; bifocal lens; contact lens; trifocal lens.

macronutrients. Substances of which the body needs large amounts to survive.

macula. The central area of the retina that is used for direct, central vision. In humans, it has only cones, no rods.

macular degeneration. Irreversible and progressive damage to the macular portion of the retina, resulting in a gradual loss of fine, or reading, vision. It is a leading cause of blindness in the United States, and is usually associated with aging.

micronutrients. Substances of which the body needs small amounts to survive.

mineral. An inorganic substance that occurs in nature. Some minerals, such as iron and calcium, are essential to the proper functioning of the human body.

motor cortex. The area of the brain that controls movement.

myopia. *See* nearsightedness.

nanometer (nm). A unit of measurement equal to one one-billionth of a meter. It is used to measure the wavelength of light.

near-vision acuity. The ability to see objects sixteen inches away or closer.

nearsightedness. A condition in which the eye is too long, the cornea too steeply curved, or the lens unable to relax, causing the light passing through the cornea to come to a focus in front of the retina when viewing a distant object; a refractive error. The nearsighted person can see near objects clearly, but sees distant objects as blurry. Also called myopia. *See also* astigmatism; emmetropia; farsightedness; presbyopia; refractive error.

oculomotor. Referring to the movement of the eyeball.

oculomotor coordination. Synchronized eye movements.

occupational progressive addition lens (OPAL). An eyeglass lens designed with no lined areas to allow clear vision at the near and intermediate viewing distances. *See also* progressive addition lens (PAL).

optometric vision therapy. A therapy program designed to realign and alter the functioning of the visual system. It includes techniques and other activities to reduce the visual stress, guide the development of the visual system, improve the visual skills, and enhance visual performance. Also called vision therapy.

peripheral vision. The part of the visual field that is outside the direct line of vision; the side vision. *See also* central vision; visual field.

photoreceptors. Sensory cells that are stimulated by light. In humans, they are the rods and cones of the retina. *See also* cones; rods.

pink eye. An inflammation of the conjunctiva. It can be caused by an infection, allergy, or irritation. Also called conjunctivitis.

polycarbonate. A type of plastic material used to make eyeglass lenses. It has a higher refractive index and more impact resistance than CR-39.

presbyopia. A condition in which the eye's lens has hardened and lost its focusing flexibility, causing difficulty with near vision; a refractive error. It usually occurs after the age of forty. *See also* astigmatism; emmetropia; farsightedness; nearsightedness; refractive error.

progressive addition lens (PAL). A type of multifocal corrective lens in which the transition from the distance segment to the intermediate segment and then to the near segment of the lens is gradual and uninterrupted. *See also* lens; trifocal lens.

protanopia. A defect in the perception of the color red. *See also* deuteranopia.

protein. A nutrient formed by a naturally occurring combination of amino acids. It is essential for growth and development.

refractive error. A condition in which the light passing through the cornea is refracted incorrectly and therefore does not come to a focus on the retina, causing blurred near and/or distance vision. *See also* astigmatism; emmetropia; farsightedness; nearsightedness; presbyopia.

retina. The inner lining of most of the back chamber of the eye. It contains layers of nerve cells that are sensitive to light.

retinol. A form of vitamin A that is found in animal tissues.

rods. The straight, thin cells in the retina of the eye. They contain rhodopsin and are responsible for night vision and vision in dim light. *See also* cones; photoreceptors.

sclera. The tough, white, fibrous outer protective layer of the eye.

scotopic sensitivity syndrome (SSS). A condition in which night vision is used at all times, which can lead to visual distortions and difficulty reading. It was first described by researcher Helen Irlen in the 1980s.

stereoscopic vision. Depth perception.

strabismus. A condition in which the two eyes do not align properly while looking at a single object. One eye turns away (out, in, up, or down) from the point of regard. *See also* crossed eyes; walleyed.

stye. A condition in which the hair follicle of an eyelash becomes infected, resulting in inflammation, redness, and soreness. *See also* chalazion.

temporal lobes. Areas of the brain located on both sides of the head surrounding the ears. The temporal lobes process auditory and some visual information.

thyroid gland. A gland located in the neck that produces thyroid hormone.

thyroid hormone. The substances produced by the thyroid gland that play a role in the regulation of the metabolism. An overabundance of thyroid hormone is associated with damage to the eyes.

thyroxine. A thyroid hormone that stimulates the conversion of carotene into a usable nutrient.

tobacco amblyopia. A loss of vision due to tobacco poisoning.

tracking. The ability to follow a moving target.

trifocal lens. A corrective lens that contains three segments—one for distance viewing, one for intermediate viewing, and one for near viewing. *See also* bifocal lens; lens.

20/20 vision. The visual acuity in the optically normal human eye. The term comes from the ability to read a specific row of letters or other symbols on a chart such as the Snellen chart from a distance of 20 feet. Deviations from the norm are expressed as, for example, 20/30, which indicates the ability to read at 20 feet what an optically normal person can read at 30 feet.

ultraviolet (UV) light. Light with a wavelength of less than 400 nanometers, which puts it below the range of the human visual spectrum.

vision therapy. *See* optometric vision therapy.

visual cortex. The part of the brain that interprets the shapes of objects and the spatial organization of scenes, and recognizes visual patterns as they belong to known objects.

visualization. The ability to form a mental image of an object that is not actually present.

vitamin. An essential organic compound necessary for human metabolism but not manufactured by the human body. Vitamins must be taken in wholly or partly from nutrient sources.

vitreous humor. A clear, jellylike substance that fills the posterior (back) chamber of the eye and serves as a support structure for the retina.

walleyed. Having an eye that turns outward while the other eye looks straight ahead. *See also* crossed eyes; strabismus.

water. An essential nutrient that is involved in every function of the body.

Resources

American Speech-Language-Hearing Association
www.asha.org
2200 Research Boulevard
Rockville, MD 20850-3289 USA
301-296-5700

Food and Nutrition Information Center
USDA ARS National Agricultural
  Library
www.nal.usda.gov/fnic
10301 Baltimore Avenue, Room 105
Beltsville, MD 20705-2351
301-504-5414

International Dyslexia Association
https://dyslexiaida.org

40 York Road, 4th Floor
Baltimore, MD 21204
410-296-0232

Irlen Institute for Perceptual and Learning Disabilities
https://irlen.com
5380 Village Road
Long Beach, CA 90808
1-800-55-IRLEN • 562-496-2550

Learning Disabilities Association of America
https://ldaamerica.org
461 Cochran Road, Suite 245
Pittsburgh, PA 15228
412-341-1515

VISION THERAPY

College of Optometrists in Vision Development
www.covd.org
info@covd.org
215 W. Garfield Rd, Ste 260
Aurora, OH 44202
330-995-0718

Eye Yoga
www.eyeyoga.com.au
31 Crudge Road
Marayong NSW 2148 (Australia)
+61 0402 857 112

**Optometric Extension Program
Foundation**
https://oepf.org

2300 York Road, Suite 113
Timonium, Maryland, 21093
410-561-3791

MISCELLANEOUS

**American Academy of
Ophthalmology**
www.aao.org
P.O. Box 7424
San Francisco, CA 94120-7424
415-561-8500

**American Academy of
Optometry**
www.aaopt.org
622 East Washington Street,
   Suite 300
Orlando, Florida 32801
844-323-EYES (3937) • 321-319-4860

American Optometric Association
www.aoa.org
243 N. Lindbergh Blvd.
St. Louis, MO 63141
800-365-2219 • 314-991-4100

College of Syntonic Optometry
https://csovision.org
csovision2020@gmail.com
2052 W. Morales Drive
Pueblo West, CO 81007
877-559-0541 • 719-547-8177

**Corporate Vision Consulting
Jeff Anshel, OD, FAAO**
www.cvconsulting.com
4624 A Kanaele Road
Kapaa, HI 96746
760-519-0024

EnChroma
https://enchroma.com
support@enchroma.com
855-323-9803

Gunnar Computer Eyewear
https://gunnar.com
support@gunnars.com
2236 Rutherford Road, Suite 123
Carlsbad, California 92008
888-486-6270

**National Academy of
Opticianry**
www.nao.org
ctucker@nao.org
8401 Corporate Drive, Suite 605
Landover, MD 20785
800-229-4828

Prevent Blindness
www.preventblindness.org
225 West Wacker Drive, Suite 400
Chicago, IL 60606
1-800-331-2020

The Vision Council
www.thevisioncouncil.org
225 Reinekers Ln, Suite 700
Alexandria, VA 22314
1-866-826-0290 • 703-548-4560

References

Chapter 1

Borish, William Benjamin. *Borish's Clinical Refraction*, 4th Ed. Philadelphia: Saunders, 1998.

Hermsen VM, Dreyer RF. "Ophthalmic anatomy." *Prim Care*. 1982 Dec;9(4): 627–45.

Grant-Kels JM, Kels BD. "Human ocular anatomy." *Dermatol Clin*. 1992 Jul;10(3): 473–82.

Iveson-Iveson J. "Anatomy and physiology: the eye." *Nurs Mirror*. 1979 Feb 22;148(8):31–3.

Chapter 2

Adams WL. "Eyestrain." *J Ky State Med Assoc*. 1957 Nov;55(11):993–6.

Duke-Elder, S. "Eyestrain." *Practitioner*. 1947 May;158(947):377–82.

De Ocampo G. "Eyestrain." *Acta Med Philipp*. 1949 Jul-Sep;6(1):9–20.

Nakamura Y. "Measurement of pupillary unrest in eyestrain." *Jpn J Ophthalmol*. 1996;40(4):533–9.

Iwasaki T, Tawara A, Miyake N. "[Effects on eyestrain of outward stimuli for accommodation]." *Nippon Ganka Gakkai Zasshi*. 2002 Oct;106(10):634–41.

Takeda T, Ostberg O, Fukui Y, et al. "Dynamic accommodation measurements for objective assessment of eyestrain and visual fatigue." *J Hum Ergol* (Tokyo). 1988 Sep;17(1):21–35.

Fishenden, RB. "Types, paper and printing in relation to eyestrain." *Br J Ophthalmol*. 1946 Jan;30:20–6.

Pimentel, PC. "[Asthenopia]." *Rev Bras Oftalmol*. 1960 Mar;19:5–10.

Hemphälä H, Eklund J. "A visual ergonomics intervention in mail sorting facilities: effects on eyes, muscles and productivity." *Appl Ergon*. 2012 Jan;43(1):217–29.

Sheedy JE, Hayes JN, Engle J. "Is all asthenopia the same?" *Optom Vis Sci*. 2003 Nov;80(11):732–9.

Abdi S, Rydberg A. "Asthenopia in schoolchildren, orthoptic and ophthalmological findings and treatment." *Doc Ophthalmol*. 2005 Sep;111(2):65–72.

Chapter 3

Long J, Cheung R, Duong S, et al. "Viewing distance and eyestrain symptoms with prolonged viewing of smartphones." *Clin Exp Optom*. 2017 Mar;100(2):133–137.

Miranda MN, García Castiñeiras S, Miranda MN Jr. "Computer eyestrain." *Bol Asoc Med P R*. 1989 Apr;81(4):137–8.

Jaiswal S, Asper L, Long J, et al. "Ocular and visual discomfort associated with smartphones, tablets and computers: what we do and do not know." *Clin Exp Optom*. 2019 Sep;102(5):463–477.

Coles-Brennan C, Sulley A, Young G. "Management of digital eyestrain." *Clin Exp Optom*. 2019 Jan;102(1):18–29.

Rosenfield M. "Computer vision syndrome: a review of ocular causes and potential treatments." *Ophthalmic Physiol Opt*. 2011 Sep;31(5):502–15.

Nakaishi H, Yamada Y. "Abnormal tear

dynamics and symptoms of eyestrain in operators of visual display terminals." *Occup Environ Med.* 1999 Jan;56(1):6–9.

Köpper M, Mayr S, Buchner A. "Reading from computer screen versus reading from paper: does it still make a difference?" *Ergonomics.* 2016 May;59(5):615–32.

Karoney MJ, Mburu SK, Ndegwa DW, et al. "Ergonomics in the computer workstation." *East Afr Med J.* 2010 Sep;87(9):382–4.

Mutti DO, Zadnik K. "Is computer use a risk factor for myopia?" *J Am Optom Assoc.* 1996 Sep;67(9):521–30.

Galinsky T, Swanson N, Sauter S, et al. "Supplementary breaks and stretching exercises for data entry operators: a follow-up field study." *Am J Ind Med.* 2007 Jul;50(7):519–27.

Jaschinski-Kruza W. "Eyestrain in VDU users: viewing distance and the resting position of ocular muscles." *Hum Factors.* 1991 Feb;33(1):69–83.

Chapter 4

Ip JM, Robaei D, Rochtchina E, Mitchell P. "Prevalence of eye disorders in young children with eyestrain complaints." *Am J Ophthalmol.* 2006 Sep;142(3):495–7.

Vesel P, Hanák L, Bene P. "Digital Eye Strain in a Population of Young Subjects." *Cesk Slov Oftalmol.* 2019 Winter;74(4):154–157.

Vilela MA, Pellanda LC, Fassa AG, et al. "Prevalence of asthenopia in children: a systematic review with meta-analysis." *J Pediatr (Rio J).* 2015 Jul-Aug;91(4):320–5.

Wilkins A. "Coloured overlays and their effects on reading speed: a review." *Ophthalmic Physiol Opt.* 2002 Sep;22(5):448–54.

Kajita M, Ono M, Suzuki S, et al. "Accommodative microfluctuation in asthenopia caused by accommodative spasm." *Fukushima J Med Sci.* 2001 Jun;47(1):13–20.

Chapter 5

Hemphälä H, Nylén P, Eklund J. "Optimal correction in spectacles: intervention effects on eyestrain and musculoskeletal discomfort among postal workers." *Work.* 2014 Jan 1;47(3):329–37.

Heus P, Verbeek JH, Tikka C. "Optical correction of refractive error for preventing and treating eye symptoms in computer users." *Cochrane Database Syst Rev.* 2018 Apr 10;4(4):CD009877.

Kee CS, Leung TW, Kan KH, Lam CH. "Effects of Progressive Addition Lens Wear on Digital Work in Pre-presbyopes." *Optom Vis Sci.* 2018 May;95(5):457–467.

Jerome B. "Vision, eyestrain, and glasses." *J Lancet.* 1960 Feb;80:48–50.

Jiménez R, Redondo B, Davies LN, Vera J. "Effects of Optical Correction Method on the Magnitude and Variability of Accommodative Response: A Test-retest Study." *Optom Vis Sci.* 2019 Aug;96(8):568–578.

Iwasaki T, Tawara A. "[Eyestrain induced by stereogram on 3-D display—differences between types of correction]." *Nippon Ganka Gakkai Zasshi.* 2002 Jul;106(7):404–10.

Papas E, Tilia D, McNally J, et al. "Ocular discomfort responses after short periods of contact lens wear." *Optom Vis Sci.* 2015 Jun;92(6):665–70.

Cagnie B, De Meulemeester K, Saeys L, et al. "The impact of different lenses on visual and musculoskeletal complaints in VDU workers with work-related neck complaints: a randomized controlled trial." *Environ Health Prev Med.* 2017 Mar 16;22(1):8.

Chapter 6

Palavets T, Rosenfield M. "Blue-blocking Filters and Digital Eyestrain." *Optom Vis Sci.* 2019 Jan;96(1):48–54.

Ide T, Toda I, Miki E, Tsubota K. "Effect of Blue Light-Reducing Eye Glasses on Critical Flicker Frequency." *Asia Pac J Ophthalmol (Phila).* 2015 Mar-Apr;4(2):80–5.

Wagle S, Kamath R, Tiwari R, et al.

"Ocular Morbidity among Students in Relation to Classroom Illumination Levels." *Indian Pediatr.* 2015 Sep;52(9):783–5.

Taylor WO. "Fluorescent lighting and eyestrain." *Practitioner.* 1977 Feb;218(1304):295–7.

Glimne S, Seimyr GÖ, Ygge J, et al. "Measuring glare induced visual fatigue by fixation disparity variation." *Work.* 2013;45(4):431–7.

Cogan DG. "Lighting, eyestrain, and health hazards." *Sight Sav Rev.* 1968 Summer;38(2):73–83.

Quarato M, Gatti MF, De Maria L, et al. "[Occupational exposure to fluorescent light in a pathologist with myopic complications and asthenopia onset]." *Med Lav.* 2017 Jun 28;108(3):228–232.

Aghemo C, Piccoli B. "[Lighting condition analysis at work]." *G Ital Med Lav Ergon.* 2004 Oct-Dec;26(4):395–400.

Chapter 7

Evans BJW, Allen PM, Wilkins AJ. "A Delphi study to develop practical diagnostic guidelines for visual stress (pattern-related visual stress)." *J Optom.* 2017 Jul-Sep;10(3):161–168.

Law TB. "Headache." *Trans Ophthalmol Soc Aust.* 1960;20:112–20.

Richter HO. "Neck pain brought into focus." *Work.* 2014 Jan 1;47(3):413–8.

Ye Z, Honda S, Abe Y, et al. "Influence of work duration or physical symptoms on mental health among Japanese visual display terminal users." *Ind Health.* 2007 Apr;45(2):328–33.

Gowrisankaran S, Nahar NK, Hayes JR, Sheedy JE. "Asthenopia and blink rate under visual and cognitive loads." *Optom Vis Sci.* 2012 Jan;89(1):97–104.

Chapter 8

Hedman LR, Briem V. "Short-term changes in eyestrain of VDU users as a function of age." *Hum Factors.* 1984 Jun;26(3):357–70.

Mónika Sztretye, Beatrix Dienes, Mónika Gönczi, et al. "Astaxanthin: A Potential Mitochondrial-Targeted Antioxidant Treatment in Diseases and with Aging." *Oxid Med Cell Longev.* 2019; 2019: 3849692.

Zimniak P. "Relationship of electrophilic stress to aging. Free Radical Biology & Medicine." 2011;51(6):1087–1105.

Rattan SI. "Theories of biological aging: genes, proteins, and free radicals." *Free Radical Research.* 2009;40(12):1230–1238.

Valko M, Leibfritz D, Moncol J, et al. "Free radicals and antioxidants in normal physiological functions and human disease." *The International Journal of Biochemistry & Cell Biology.* 2007;39(1):44–84.

Chapter 9

Maeda-Yamamoto M, Nishimura M, Kitaichi N, et al. "A Randomized, Placebo-Controlled Study on the Safety and Efficacy of Daily Ingestion of Green Tea (Camellia sinensis L.) cv. "Yabukita" and "Sunrouge" on Eyestrain and Blood Pressure in Healthy Adults." *Nutrients.* 2018 May 6;10(5):569.

Ozawa Y, Kawashima M, Inoue S, et al. "Bilberry extract supplementation for preventing eye fatigue in video display terminal workers." *J Nutr Health Aging.* 2015 May;19(5):548–54.

Keiko Kono, Yoshiki Shimizu, Satomi Takahashi, et al. "Effect of Multiple Dietary Supplement Containing Lutein, Astaxanthin, Cyanidin-3-Glucoside, and DHA on Accommodative Ability." *Curr Med Chem.* 2014 Aug; 14(2): 114–125.

Fusco D, Colloca G, Lo Monaco MR, et al. "Effects of antioxidant supplementation on the aging process." *Clinical Interventions in Aging.* 2007;2(3):377–387.

Ghazi Hussein, Ushio Sankawa, Hirozo Goto, et al. "Astaxanthin, a carotenoid with potential in human health and nutrition." *Nat Prod* 2006 Mar;69(3):443–9.

Giannaccare G, Pellegrini M, Senni C, et al. "Clinical Applications of Astaxanthin in the Treatment of Ocular Diseases: Emerging Insights." *Mar Drugs*. 2020 May 1;18(5):239.

Gaby AR. "Nutritional therapies for ocular disorders: Part Three." *Altern Med Rev*. 2008 Sep;13(3):191–204.

Kawabata F, Tsuji T. "Effects of dietary supplementation with a combination of fish oil, bilberry extract, and lutein on subjective symptoms of asthenopia in humans." *Biomed Res*. 2011 Dec;32(6):387–93.

Nakaishi H, Matsumoto H, Tominaga S, et al. "Effects of black current anthocyanoside intake on dark adaptation and VDT work-induced transient refractive alteration in healthy humans." *Altern Med Rev*. 2000 Dec;5(6):553–62.

Chapter 10

Nakaishi H, Yamada Y. "Abnormal tear dynamics and symptoms of eyestrain in operators of visual display terminals." *Occup Environ Med*. 1999 Jan;56(1):6–9.

Katsuyama I, Arakawa T. "A novel in vitro model for screening and evaluation of anti-asthenopia drugs." *J Pharmacol Sci*. 2003 Oct;93(2):222–4.

Han MH, Craig SB, Rutner D, et al. "Medications prescribed to brain injury patients: a retrospective analysis." *Optometry*. 2008 May;79(5):252–8.

Dralands L, Garin P. "[Harmful effects of common drugs on the visual apparatus. Anti-infective drugs. A. Antibacterial agents]." *Bull Soc Belge Ophtalmol*. 1972;160(1):326–89.

Physicians' Desk Reference 2003, 57th Ed. Thomson PDR, 2002.

Andre Farkouh, Peter Frigo, and Martin Czejka1. "Systemic side effects of eye drops: a pharmacokinetic perspective." *Clin Ophthalmol*. 2016; 10: 2433–2441.

Marmor MF, et al. "Recommendations on screening for chloroquine and hydroxychloroquine retinopathy (2016 revision)." *Ophthalmology*. 2016;123: 1386–1394.

Chapter 11

Eyles M. "Functional home exercises in cases of eyestrain." *Am J Ophthalmol*. 1948 Jan;31(1):45–8.

Lavrich JB. "Convergence insufficiency and its current treatment." *Curr Opin Ophthalmol*. 2010 Sep;21(5):356–60.

Feng Y, Wang L, Chen F. "An Eye-tracking based Evaluation on the Effect of Far-infrared Therapy for Relieving Visual Fatigue." *Annu Int Conf IEEE Eng Med Biol Soc*. 2019 Jul;2019:313–316.

London R, Crelier RS. "Fixation disparity analysis: sensory and motor approaches." *Optometry*. 2006 Dec;77(12):590–608.

Smith W. "Asthenopia and orthoptics." *Am J Optom Arch Am Acad Optom*. 1961 Nov;38:637–45.

Singman EL, Matta NS, Silbert DI. "Convergence insufficiency associated with migraine: a case series." *Am Orthopt J*. 2014;64:112–6.

Brinkley JR Jr, Walonker F. "Convergence amplitude insufficiency." *Ann Ophthalmol*. 1983 Sep;15(9):826–8, 830–1.

Moore S. "The accommodative effort syndrome." *Am Orthopt J*. 1967;17:5–7.

Omori M, Watanabe T, Takai J, et al. "An attempt at preventing asthenopia among VDT workers." *Int J Occup Saf Ergon*. 2003;9(4):453–62.

Chase C, Tosha C, Borsting E, et al. "Visual discomfort and objective measures of static accommodation." *Optom Vis Sci*. 2009 Jul;86(7):883–9.

Cooper J, Feldman J, Selenow A, et al. "Reduction of asthenopia after accommodative facility training." *Am J Optom Physiol Opt*. 1987 Jun;64(6):430–6.

About the Author

Jeffrey R. Anshel, OD, received his Bachelor of Science degree in visual science and his Doctorate of Optometry from the Illinois College of Optometry. After his service in the US Navy, Dr. Anshel went into private practice, offering his patients nutrition and alternative therapies as part of their vision care. Dr. Anshel is the creator of the "20-20-20" rule for computer display users. He lectures internationally and has written eight books on eye care, including *Smart Medicine for Your Eyes* and *What You Must Know About Age-Related Macular Degeneration.* Dr. Anshel currently lives in Kauai, Hawaii.

Index

OTHER SQUAREONE TITLES OF INTEREST

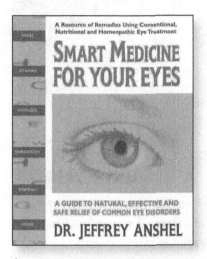

Smart Medicine for Your Eyes

A Guide to Natural, Effective, and Safe Relief of Common Eye Disorders
Jeffrey Anshel, OD

Trouble can start with headaches, blurred vision, and difficulty seeing at night. Certainly, going to an eye-care professional for help is essential, but to be part of the solution, you must also be informed. That's why *Smart Medicine for Your Eyes* was written. Here is an A-to-Z guide to the most common eye disorders and their treatments, using both conventional and alternative care.

Written in an easy-to-understand style, *Smart Medicine* is divided into three parts. Part One provides a simple overview of how the eyes work. It also clearly explains various treatment methods foe eye problems, including herbal, homeopathic, and nutritional therapies; acupressure; and acupuncture. A useful section on choosing the eye-care specialist best suited to handle your particular problem helps guide you to appropriate professional care. Part Two is a comprehensive A-to-Z directory to childhood and adult eye disorders and their various treatment options. Finally, Part Three guides you in using the specific techniques and procedures suggested in Part Two. Handy troubleshooting and first-aid sections are highlighted throughout for quick reference.

A vital bridge between the best of mainstream medicine and proven traditional therapies, *Smart Medicine for Your Eyes* is a reliable source of information that you can turn to time and time again to protect the greatest of your possessions—your eyes.

$19.95 US / $28.95 CAN • 432 pages • 7.5 x 9-inch paperback • ISBN 978-0-7570-0301-1

What You Must Know About Dry Eye

How to Prevent, Stop, or Reverse Dry Eye Disease

Jeffrey Anshel, OD

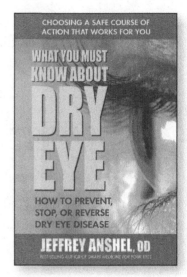

While the condition known as dry eye may sound like a minor problem, it can cause tremendous discomfort, even pain. Worse, this disorder can lead to eye fatigue, blurred vision, and difficulty driving, especially at night. In a healthy eye, lubricating tears continuously bathe the cornea—the dome-shaped outer surface of the eye. These tears provide a layer of liquid protection from the environment while nourishing the cells, keeping the eyes comfortable, and helping the eyes function properly. But when the glands near the eyes fail to produce tears of adequate quality or quantity, dry eye disease occurs.

Written by optometrist Jeffrey Anshel, *What You Must Know About Dry Eye* is divided into two parts. Part One begins by explaining the anatomy of the eye and how it works. It then focuses on dry eye—what the condition is, what causes it, how it impacts vision, and how it is diagnosed. In Part Two, the author examines a full range of treatments. First, he looks at conventional therapies, from over-the-counter artificial tears to prescription drugs. He then guides the reader in using smart nutrition and a proven supplement plan to relieve dry eye while making the eyes healthier, more comfortable, and able to see more clearly.

If you are one of the millions of people who suffer from dry eye, you know that this disorder can affect both your feeling of well-being and your ability to function in the world. *What You Must Know About Dry Eye* tells you how to relieve this common condition while improving and safeguarding your vision.

$16.95 US / $23.95 CAN • 144 pages • 6 x 9-inch paperback • ISBN 978-0-7570-0479-7

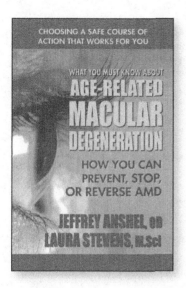

CHOOSING A SAFE COURSE OF
ACTION THAT WORKS FOR YOU

WHAT YOU MUST KNOW ABOUT
AGE-RELATED
MACULAR
DEGENERATION
HOW YOU CAN
PREVENT, STOP,
OR REVERSE AMD

JEFFREY ANSHEL, OD
LAURA STEVENS, M.Sci

What You Must Know About Age-Related Macular Degeneration

How You Can Prevent, Stop, or Reverse AMD

Jeffrey Anshel, OD,
and Laura Stevens, M.Sci

Age-related macular degeneration—AMD—is the most commonly diagnosed eye disorder in people over fifty. Well over two million Americans have been told they have AMD, and that number is expected to grow substantially. While this is a frightening statistic, over the last several years, medical researchers have shown that a number of effective treatments can slow, stop, or even reverse the progress of AMD. Now, bestselling authors Dr. Jeffrey Anshel and Laura Stevens, who herself has been diagnosed with this condition, have joined forces to produce an up-to-date guide to what you need to know to combat or even prevent AMD.

The book is divided into four parts. Part One explains how the eye works and how AMD develops, in both its wet and its dry forms. It then looks at the most common risk factors and explains how each of these factors negatively affects the structures of the eye. In Part Two, the authors look at the specific nutrients that affect the various cells of the eye. Included is a discussion of AREDS—the National Eye Institute's study that showed which supplements help protect the eye from disease. Part Three offers an additional weapon against AMD: diet. It explains why diet matters and offers advice on selecting foods that promote eye health while eliminating those that do the most damage. Part Four provides practical suggestions and easy-to-follow tips on how to incorporate this valuable information into your life.

If AMD runs in your family or you have been diagnosed with this potentially life-altering condition, it is important to know that there is not only hope, but a real path to a better, healthier life. Knowledge is power, and the more you know, the more likely you are to avoid the consequences of AMD. Let *What You Must Know About Age-Related Macular Degeneration* help you safeguard one of your most precious gifts—eyesight.

$17.95 US / $25.95 CAN • 288 pages • 6 x 9-inch paperback • ISBN 978-0-7570-0449-0

What You Must Know About Food and Supplements for Optimal Vision Care

Ocular Nutrition Handbook
Jeffrey Anshel, OD

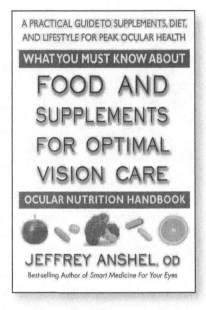

As children, we were told to eat our carrots if we wanted good eyesight. Carrots contain beta-carotene, which the body can convert into vitamin A—a necessary nutrient for optimal vision. For most of us, that's where our knowledge of vitamins and eye health stops. Over the last twenty years, many studies have demonstrated that certain foods and natural supplements can play a major role in the treatment of eye problems. From the bestselling author of *Smart Medicine for Your Eyes* comes a concise guide to these powerful substances.

What You Must Know About Food and Supplements for Optimal Vision Care is divided into three parts. Part One is an overview of nutritional principles. This section explores the function of nutrients that benefit not only the visual system but also the entire body. Part Two provides a list of common eye disorders and includes a brief discussion of each condition, supplying handy charts that detail the nutritional, herbal, and homeopathic treatments that may be used to alleviate each disorder. Part Three offers further guidance by presenting dietary approaches to eye health and providing important information on the interaction of various foods and medications.

By eating mindfully and choosing supplements wisely, there is much you can do to support eye health. In this helpful and easy-to-use resource, Dr. Anshel provides you with a wealth of information on the most effective natural products and foods available to promote optimal vision.

$16.95 US / $23.95 CAN • 176 pages • 6 x 9-inch paperback • ISBN 978-0-7570-0410-0

High Performance Vision

How to Improve Your Visual Acuity, Hone Your Motor Skills & Up Your Game

Dr. Donald S. Teig

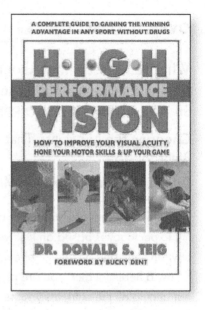

Beyond physical superiority, mental stamina, and good instincts, most of the world's best athletes possess another specific advantage that gives them an edge. We're not talking about performance-enhancing drugs, but rather something a lot simpler: good vision. Being able to follow a fastball as it flies over home plate, judge the shooting distance to a basketball hoop, or catch a spiraling football at just the right moment all depend on having good eyesight. The ability to maximize your vision can mean the difference between being a good player and a great one. In his new book, *High Performance Vision*, sports-vision specialist Dr. Donald S. Teig shares his highly successful approach to visual enhancement.

Part One includes a questionnaire to help you determine your athletic goals, gives a brief overview of the visual system, and explores the many eye conditions and injuries common to athletes. It also describes the ways in which eyesight may be measured and lists available corrective options. But *High Performance Vision* is about much more than simply correcting your vision. Part Two goes on to explain how this training program can optimize your eyesight and allow you to reach new heights of athletic success. It outlines both at-home and in-office eye exercises to help achieve peak vision.

If you've been looking for a safe, natural way to improve your game, *High Performance Vision* offers the perfect solution. In a clear and reader-friendly style, it shows you how to attain the edge you've been missing. Whether you are a weekend warrior, little leaguer, or elite athlete, this book is for you!

$17.95 US / $25.95 CAN • 176 pages • 6 x 9-inch paperback • ISBN 978-0-7570-0399-8

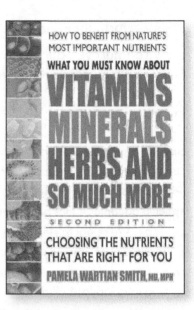